Safety And Techniques In Perfusion

Charles C. Reed

Chief Emeritus,
Perfusion Technology Section,
Texas Heart Institute,
Houston, Texas.

Mark Kurusz

Chief Perfusionist,
Clinical Instructor,
Department of Surgery,
The University of Texas Medical Branch,
Galveston, Texas.

A. Earl Lawrence, Jr.

Chief Perfusionist, Retired
Executive Director, Retired
The Alabama Heart Institute,
Birmingham, Alabama.

Quali-Med, Inc.
Stafford, Texas 1988

Printed in the United States of America

Library of Congress Cataloging In Publication Data

Reed, Charles C., 1936—
Safety and techniques in perfusion.
Includes bibliographies and index.
1. Heart, Mechanical — Safety measures.
2. Cardiopulmonary bypass.
I. Kurusz, Mark, 1946.
II. Lawrence, A. Earl, 1946.
III. Title.
[DNLM: 1. Cardiopulmonary bypass — methods.
2. Perfusion — methods. WG 168 R333s]
RD598.35.M42R44 1988 617'.412 88-61551

ISBN 0-929511-00-X

Foreword

Samuel Johnson in 1777 wrote "Depend upon it, sir, when a man knows he is to be hanged in a fortnight, it concentrates his mind wonderfully."Paraphrased for 1988 his thought could read "Nothing so focuses the mind on issues of safety as the prospect of a malpractice suit." For those not yet mind-focused by a malpractice suit, the lawsuits and case notes in these chapters should provide perfusionists with the motivation to regard safety as their prime responsibility.

At first glance it would seem that governmental agencies well protect, even over-protect, the public in issues of safety. Before introduction of any new drug, federal law requires extensive toxicological and teratogenic testing. Every new medical device for diagnosis or treatment must survive safety testing before release for patient use. In addition many hospitals conduct their own safety testing on devices already warranted as safe by manufacturers and approved by government regulatory agencies. These measures are effective and prevent untoward events or accidents for which tests are available, that is, those **which can be anticipated.** Ultimate safety however, can be known only after a drug or device has been extensively used in the population at large. Postmarketing surveillance of use in millions of patients representing all population variants, all diseases and the entire spectrum of indications is the only methods which uncovers unanticipated drug toxicity or misuse and failures of devices. Only this method reveals adverse effects and accidents **which were not anticipated**, not tested for and discovers a true estimate of safety.

Prevention of rare events is a generic problem not limited to medicine. Airplane and auto manufacturers build in safety features designed to prevent any accident which occurred in the past by a known mechanism. No safety features can be included to prevent accidents by mechanisms not even imagined. Compared to 30 years ago, perfusion has become extraordinarily safe, in part because of the many safety features built into the equipment based on accidents of the past. Despite this, accidents continue to occur with disastrous patient outcomes. Are these disasters simply from inattention, complacency and lack of vigilance? Or are they from perfusionists' extraordinary ingenuity in finding new ways to misuse equipment? Or perhaps the infinite variations with which surgeons perform and patients respond provide the rare opportunities for disaster? Is it all of these?

A continuous surveillance of the outcomes of all perfusions can identify bad results and with good documentation, can identify causes. With known cause, a preventive remedy can be devised. This is the ideal way, logical but tactically almost impossible. Failing this, prevention of rare accidents requires anticipation of accidents by all theoretically possible mechanisms and by analysis of all accidents which have occurred. This is what this book is all about. For safety, every perfusion no matter how simple or brief must incorporate techniques effective in preventing both common and rare disasters.

The authors' collective experience and wisdom in perfusion technology is awesome. In addition to their own experience they have ranged widely among their colleagues to bring together a collection of bad outcomes and their best thoughts on prevention by awareness and by use of safety oriented techniques. Despite all the controversial aspects as to what constitutes optimal perfusion one aspect of perfusion technology is not debatable - the overwhelmingly prime responsibility of the perfusionist is the prevention of accidents. If this book serves to "concentrate the mind wonderfully" on the prime importance of safety in perfusion, it will have benefited a generation of patients.

Arthur S. Keats, M.D.
Division of Cardiovascular Anesthesia
Texas Heart Institute
Houston, Texas

Preface

Since its inception, during the year Napoleon led the Grand Army to Moscow and the Anglo-American war was raging over freedom on the high seas, cardiopulmonary bypass has made quantum leaps in some areas while in others it is hesitantly creeping out of the cave in search of fire. Science has been defined as "the systematic classification of experience." Perfusion today is far from having enough experience to be thought of as a science. Science exists in perfusion to be sure, but the perfusionist must provide a significant amount of art to routine cardiopulmonary bypass to bring about a satisfactory outcome. Emergencies occurring during perfusion require even more art from the perfusionist as well as experience and deductive reasoning for a successful result. Art is more difficult to define. It is composed of technique, in large part, and of experience, reasoning, and a part that is indefinable. Some problems which confounded early investigators are as equally perplexing today. Other problems have vanished from the literature without ever having been satisfactorily explained and perhaps now should be referred to as non-problems. One wonders which of today's unsolved and unreconciled controversies will be tomorrow's non-problems.

As the techniques of cardiopulmonary bypass have evolved and the educational process of the perfusionist has developed, the availability of literature for the perfusionist and others interested in cardiopulmonary bypass has lagged far behind. "Technique" books have been written by physicians for physicians. Certainly selected aspects of these books are of interest and are educational to the perfusionist, but much esoterica is included that is far outside the areas of interest, responsibilities, or effective response of the clinical perfusionist.

The one failing of all available books is in the area of safety during cardiopulmonary bypass. One of the authors recently conducted a benchmark perfusion safety survey of the clinical perfusion community, and much of the data contained therein is referenced in this book. To avoid repetitive footnoting we have referred to this information, where included, simply as The Survey.*

Another common failing of the available books is in explaining, from a practical standpoint, how the procedure should be done, what type of circuit is needed, what the perfusion parameters should be, what are the dangers and pitfalls of the technique.

In this book we have attempted to fill both voids by including normal and advanced techniques in cardiopulmonary bypass and addressing both from the standpoint of safety or by describing, in our opinion, the safest methodology that may be employed.

It is the authors' hope that perfusion students, clinical perfusionists, and all others concerned with or interested in perfusion will find the book beneficial and thought-provoking.

Included at the end of most chapters is a section entitled ..LAWSUITS AND ...CASENOTES. The Lawsuits described are ones in which the authors had direct knowledge. The Casenotes include comments from The Survey, personal experiences of the authors, and anecdotal experiences of our colleagues. Their inclusion serves to emphasize points of safe perfusion practice included in that chapter although many are appropriate for inclusion in several chapters. Others may appear to be included in more than one chapter. They are not.

*Kurusz M, Conti VR, Arens JF, Brown JP, Faulkner SC, Manning Jr JV: Perfusion accident survey. Proceed Am Acad Cardiovasc Perfusion 7:57-65, 1986.

It is simply that the specific type of accident has happened on more than one occasion, and regrettably, sometimes on several or many occasions.

It is also the hope of these authors that confrontation with the stark reality of what has happened before and what can happen again will have a deterrent effect on complacent perfusion practices. Techniques and practices must be constantly re-evaluated in the cold harsh light of safety and adequacy of perfusion. Just because the perfusionist has "gotten by" with a particular technique repeatedly does not demonstrate that the technique is safe or effective. The disaster from a fatal flaw in the technique can be looming just around the corner of the next case. The days of "don't change a thing if it works" are long past. To persist in this thinking is to invite a catastrophic perfusion accident and possibly subsequent devastating malpractice lawsuit.

Charles C. Reed

Mark Kurusz

A. Earl Lawrence, Jr.

Pickle's Gap 1988

CONTENTS

Chapter 1:

PERFUSIONIST DUTIES AND RESPONSIBILITIES

Chapter 1: PERFUSIONIST DUTIES AND RESPONSIBILITIES

Over the past ten years there has been much discussion, with little resolution, regarding the duties, responsibilities, and sphere of influence of the perfusionist. Once special interests and unique situations are set aside, the duties and responsibilities of the perfusionist become rather clear cut. **A duty is that which one is bound to do, or not do, by moral or legal obligation.** A duty carries with it, and in part is circumferentially defined by, responsibilities directly related to that duty. **Responsibilities are things which one is answerable or accountable for because they are within one's power of choice or control or under one's management or care.**[1]

1. The primary duty of a perfusionist is the operation of the heart-lung machine to provide cardiovascular support for a patient undergoing cardiac or non-cardiac surgery. The primary responsibility associated with this duty is the safety of the patient undergoing such a procedure. The number one safety hazard accompanying this activity has always been, and continues to be, the introduction of air into a patient's cardiovascular system. The primary source of such introduction of air into the cardiovascular system, by the perfusionist, is that of pumping micro or macro air emboli from the cardiopulmonary bypass circuit. The oxygenating devices in use today continue to be produced in the original designs. The medical device industry is apparently unable to design them in such a way as to make the hazard of air embolism impossible. Therefore, it remains *the ultimate and primary responsibility of the cardiovascular perfusionist to not allow the oxygenating device be emptied thereby introducing air into the cardiovascular system of the patient.*

This description, at first glance, appears to be a negative or reactive type activity on the part of the perfusionist. At closer look, and with more experience in the field of perfusion, it is very clear that this is not the case at all. This is an extremely active endeavor on the part of the perfusionist and the other members of the open-heart surgery team. This activity involves first, and above all, essential and effective communication among each of the teams involved in the open-heart surgery procedure (see Chapter 3: INTERFACE). The perfusionist must consider this primary hazard uppermost in their attention in all activities during an open-heart surgery procedure, and in all communications with others involved. Air may be introduced into the system in a wide variety of ways (see Chapter 26: AIR) and it is the responsibility of everyone involved to keep this possibility in the forefront of their thinking during a cardiopulmonary bypass procedure.

Safety must be the overriding consideration in a perfusion case regardless of all mechanical or other duties and responsibilities with which the perfusionists may be engaged. Although others may have accepted the responsibility for supervision and control of the perfusion procedure, the perfusionist must assist them in maintaining a safe environment for the patient undergoing cardiopulmonary bypass.[2]

The perfusionist is responsible for maintaining the sterility and integrity of the bypass circuit at all times during assembly and operation. This includes verification of the sterility and integrity of packaging of disposable equipment used. The perfusionist is further responsible for the protection against any damage to the circuit by any individuals during the assembly or use during the procedure. Proper disposal of all disposable items used by the perfusionist is also their responsibility. This includes any and all used tubing, reservoirs, oxygenators, or blood immediately following completion of a case, as well as the proper cleaning all permanent equipment after use.

2. It is the duty of the perfusionist to maintain adequate blood flow for the patient undergoing cardiovascular perfusion. The responsibilities involved in this duty include calculation of the proper blood flow necessary according to protocol, and maintaining that flow throughout the bypass procedure and reacting to and adjusting the blood flow in response to hemodynamic or metabolic changes resulting from other activities occurring during the procedure. Should clinical parameters dictate that the calculated blood flow is too little or too great it is the responsibility of the perfusionist to adjust this flow accordingly, to maintain homeostasis.

3. It is the duty of the perfusionist to maintain an adequate blood pressure for the patient during cardiopulmonary bypass within the limitations of the cardiopulmonary bypass circuit and procedure. The responsibility of the perfusionist is to maintain and regulate that blood pressure in accordance with accepted standards, and as always, in communication with the other members of the open-heart surgery team.

4. It is the duty of the perfusionist to maintain adequate oxygenation of the blood during cardiopulmonary bypass. The responsibilities of the perfusionist include assessing the patient's preexisting condition and type of surgery scheduled in order to choose the proper device to be used for oxygenation during cardiopulmonary bypass, in consultation with the surgeon/physician in charge. Further responsibilities include operation of this device, in accordance with the manufacturer's printed instructions, to maintain normal or adequate blood gas status during the perfusion procedure. This responsibility includes adjusting to changes in the condition of the patient during the procedure and continuing to maintain adequate oxygenation and removal of carbon dioxide, at a normal base excess (see Chapter 15: ACID-BASE BALANCE).

5. It is the duty of the perfusionist to operate suction pumps and devices that remove blood from the operative field or vent various chambers of the heart. This additional responsibility of a perfusionist presents a further demand to effectively communicate with the other members of the team. Needle-vent evacuation of air from various cardiac chambers and great vessels also is utilized during open and non-open-heart surgery procedures usually on a routine basis. The suction applied to a needle or aspiration vent placed into a cardiac chamber requires constant and direct communication between the surgeon and the perfusionist in order to avoid introduction of air into the cardiac chambers, or ineffective venting, thus negating the original intention of the procedure, evacuation of air or blood. Maintaining adequate decompression of various chambers of the heart is an extremely important responsibility and one in which the perfusionist must assist the surgeon to the best of their ability. The use of an intra-cardiac or extra-cardiac suction device also presents the perfusionist with the responsibility of understanding the significance of blood trauma caused by these devices, and a responsibility to regulate this suction in as gentle manner as possible to keep hemolysis at an absolute minimum.

6. The maintenance and regulation of the blood temperature, and thereby the body temperature, of the patient undergoing cardiopulmonary bypass is the duty of the cardiovascular perfusionist. Desired blood and organ temperature is variable according to the procedure, institution, and surgeon in charge, in which open-heart surgery is practiced. The safe use of an adequate temperature gradient when both cooling and rewarming is the responsibility of the perfusionist. The safety of and accuracy of devices used to accomplish this duty is the responsibility of the perfusionist (see Chapter 16: HYPOTHERMIA).

7. It is the duty of the perfusionist to record all relevant perfusion information during cardiopulmonary bypass, and maintain such records in accordance with the practice and policy of their institution. Perfusion records vary from hospital to hospital, but it is the responsibility of the perfusionist to understand their local situation and conform to the policies of the institution in which they practice to ensure that adequate basic information is recorded (see Chapter 5: CHARTING). Such records provide valuable follow-up information should any questions arise at a later date, as well as providing a continuous learning experience for the perfusionist. In the event of a patient injury, information is often required at a much later date in order to adequately prove the efficacy of one's judgment.

8. Preventive maintenance of all equipment used by the perfusionist, and records of such maintenance, is the duty of the perfusionist. Under duties of an individual so dependent upon mechanical equipment for the accomplishment of the demanding task of perfusion, it almost seems unnecessary to mention the responsibility of preventive maintenance. However, a review of court cases demonstrates very little compliance with this obvious responsibility. Therefore it is a responsibility that preventive maintenance should be performed, at least once every six months, or more frequently if recommended by the manufacturer or institutional guidelines, of all equipment used to accomplish the duties of the perfusionist. It is the responsibility of the perfusionist to keep records of routine maintenance, preventive maintenance, and inspections of all perfusion-related equipment. These records must be kept for at least six years. Preventive maintenance includes pre-bypass calibration of any and all devices used by the perfusionist.

9. It is the duty of the perfusionist to practice acceptable standards in their practice of perfusion. These standards may be specific to an individual surgeon's protocol, institutional standards or policy, or may be national or regional in nature. For example, one surgeon may require a range of arterial pressure that they wish to have maintained during bypass, while another surgeon may have another set of values to maintain during his cases. The perfusionist has the responsibility to operate within the responsible surgeon's stated protocol. Institutional standards may involve preventive maintenance of equipment or sterility requirements. National standards involve the certification process and continuing education, as well as published standards of practice. Additionally it is a duty and responsibility of the perfusionist to maintain adequate records of the performance of their activities and professional performance.

10. Other duties require the performance of perfusion activities upon order or direction. That is, the perfusionist must be available in their own particular situation to supply their services in accordance with the needs of the patient.

Additional Duties and Responsibilities

It is a professional responsibility of the perfusionist to maintain their continuing education and current knowledge of the practice of perfusion. It is a further responsibility of the perfusionist to share their knowledge and experience, not only with the professional community, but also within their own institution, and certainly with the other teams that are involved in the performance of open-heart surgery. As one accepts professional duties, one must accept professional responsibilities. This includes the implied contract between that professional and the general public who requires their services. These professional responsibilities require subscription to a code of ethics in the performance of all activities.

It is quite natural, as new procedures are initiated and new devices to perform these procedures are developed, that the surgeon/physician in charge of the operating room would look to the individual, or individuals, they feel most competent and responsible to operate these devices. However, one must remember that any additional duties added to a perfusionist will by necessity take time, energy, concentration, and effort away from other activities. It is the belief of these authors that if any additional devices, other than those that are included in the duties of the perfusionist, are utilized, additional manpower is necessary so as not to detract from the primary duties and responsibilities of the perfusionist during cardiopulmonary bypass.

If one decides to accept other duties or is forced to accept other duties, that may or may not detract from their primary duties and responsibilities, they must be willing to accept the additional responsibilities that accompany those duties or resist the additions vigorously.

REFERENCES

1. *Standard Dictionary of the English Language*. New York: Funk and Wagnalls, 1974.
2. Statement on extracorporeal technology. J Thorac Cardiovasc Surg 79:316, 1980.

..LAWSUITS AND ...CASENOTES

.. After approximately one hour of cardiopulmonary bypass for a three vessel coronary bypass operation, and upon release of the aortic cross- clamp, the surgeon remarked that the heart immediately went into a contracted rigorous state. He further remarked that the heart and chest wall seemed very warm. The measured esophageal temperature was 47°C. Upon examination it was obvious that the patient had multiple organ system damage from hyperthermia. The patient was pronounced dead and a lawsuit ensued.

The hot and cold water lines leading to the heart-lung machine had been reversed during connection to the pump by a perfusion assistant. Throughout the weeks of questioning the perfusionist insisted that he was not responsible for the accident, and that he was not responsible for the monitoring of the patient's temperature. The primary perfusionist is responsible for the operation of the heart-lung machine during open-heart surgery, and if one chooses to use perfusion assistants then they are responsible for the perfusion assistant's conduct as well.

The case was settled out of court for $500,000 with financial liability divided between the surgeon, the insurer for the hospital (perfusionist), and the manufacturer of the heart-lung machine.

STANDARDS OF PRACTICE

Adopted September 21, 1987*

The American Academy of Cardiovascular Perfusion acknowledges and concurs that the primary responsibility for the care of the patient undergoing procedures involving cardiopulmonary bypass rests with Surgeon/Physician in charge. The Academy believes that it is the responsibility of the perfusionist to assist the Surgeon/Physician in any way possible in this patient care, and particularly within the defined area of expertise of the perfusionist, that of cardiopulmonary bypass equipment, ancillary equipment, and procedures. The American Academy of Cardiovascular Perfusion endorses the following standards of practice in the art of Cardiopulmonary Bypass, and acknowledges that the development of standards of practice is an ongoing process due to evolving technology.

RECORDS. A written perfusion record must be kept of each procedure, and must include pertinent direct or indirect patient information during the procedure e.g., medical record number, age, weight, important preexisting conditions, diagnosis, equipment used including serial and/or lot numbers. Drugs and fluids added through either the prime or bypass circuit during the procedure must be upon the prescription of a physician, and time and amounts recorded as part of the record. Perfusion parameters must be recorded at no less than every 15 minutes or whenever one of the parameters is changed or changes, whichever is shorter.

Perfusion parameters that must be recorded (but not limited to) are: time; flow rate; perfusion pressure; temperature; perfusion gas mixtures and flow rates. Blood gases must be recorded when obtained, and any other pertinent information (e.g., drugs added, fluid added, instructions regarding changes to flow, cooling and rewarming). A copy of the perfusion record must be retained by the perfusionist. A copy should be placed in the patient chart if that is within the particular hospital rules and regulations. This record should contain all other information pertinent to the bypass procedure.

EQUIPMENT. Although the weight of the patient, preexisting conditions and the selected procedure will dictate certain aspects of the selection of equipment, other aspects of equipment selection are not so affected. The perfusionist should make genuine efforts at cost containment through the various methods available to them. However, optimal performance and safety of the perfusion circuit is the prime concern of the perfusionist. Perfusionists must utilize safety equipment currently available in the selection of the perfusion circuit (e.g., low level alarm sensors, bubble detectors, bubble traps, automatic shutoff devices, arterial line filters, and others deemed appropriate for safety). Suction and vent lines must be tested immediately prior to use. Permanent equipment must have periodic scheduled preventive maintenance, and records of such maintenance must be kept by the perfusionist. The perfusionist should consult with the Surgeon/Physician in charge of the procedure regarding equipment.

*Reprinted by permission of The American Academy of Cardiovascular Perfusion.

PERSONNEL. Two qualified perfusionists are preferable during a cardiopulmonary bypass procedure. If the primary perfusionist is required to do more than operate the heart-lung machine, including the cardiopulmonary bypass circuit, and perform manipulations with this circuit (e.g., draw blood gas samples and add drugs on prescription) then the perfusionist must have a qualified assistant present.

PREBYPASS. A prebypass check list must be employed. This list should include, but not be limited to, evaluation of, e.g., mixing valve, flow meters, RPM gauges, pressure monitors, direction of intended flow in tubing through the pumphead, connections, safety devices, temperature probes, and general integrity and security of the cardiopulmonary bypass system. Initial heparin dose and time must be verified and should be recorded.

PERFUSION. During cardiopulmonary bypass, an adequately safe volume must be maintained in the perfusion circuit. This volume of fluid should permit a reaction time of at least 15 seconds should venous return be interrupted. Perfusion flow rate must be maintained at such a level that inadequate tissue perfusion is not permitted (e.g., increasing metabolic acidosis, venous desaturation, EEG changes). Perfusion pressure must be maintained at an adequate level so that organ preservation and function are not compromised or impaired function detected. Anticoagulation assessment must be performed on a routine basis during cardiopulmonary bypass, and must be included as part of the perfusion record. Anticoagulation should be adequate to prevent clotting in the extracorporeal circuit and consumption of clotting factors. During the time that the heart-lung machine is not being used actively to transfuse or support the patient, both the arterial and venous lines must be securely clamped.

GENERAL. The Academy encourages the perfusionist to take an active role, in consultation with the Surgeon/Physician in charge, in developing patient contact. It is through this personal contact that promotion of responsibility and accountability of perfusion services is developed. Each patient is an individual whose preexisting clinical condition and disease dictates specific cardiopulmonary bypass considerations. A thorough knowledge and understanding of the patient's medical history through study of the medical record must be developed.

While this statement is not wholly inclusive, it represents a statement of recommendations that must be carefully considered by the cardiovascular perfusionist. This statement will be periodically updated to represent the current status of recommended standards of practice.

Chapter 2:

LEGAL AND RISK MANAGEMENT FOR PERFUSIONISTS

Chapter 2: LEGAL AND RISK MANAGEMENT FOR PERFUSIONISTS

Risk management has been defined by many different authors, and most definitions deal with the control of financial losses.[1-3] Since the word "risk" has a negative connotation and "management" is considered an active or positive activity, there seems to be a contradiction in terms, at first glance. However, one of the more appropriate definitions of risk management is presented as "a positive activity to avoid negative results."[4] The authors believe it is very appropriate, in a book on techniques in perfusion, to present for consideration some positive techniques that perhaps would enable the reader to avoid negative outcomes.

Job Description

One of the more frequently asked questions from perfusionists is, *"What can I do to prepare for a Lawsuit?"* The answer is that preparation for litigation begins long before a lawsuit or malpractice litigation is initiated. The conscientious perfusionist should begin this preparation simultaneously with beginning their employment as a perfusionist.

Certainly one of the most important parts of beginning employment, regardless of the employer, is the establishment of a job description. Every employer should require a new employee to either review an existing job description or write the duties that one will be responsible for performing. This is an activity that must be performed initially and periodically, and the perfusionist should seize the opportunity to benefit from it, both in the present and the future.

A job description should contain all of the activities that one is expected to perform, both with and without direct supervision. This job description should then be reviewed, approved, and signed, by everyone involved in direct and indirect supervision. The job description then should be approved at the highest possible administrative level within the organization, including even the hospital Board of Directors. The job description becomes the ground rules under which an individual can operate or function. By having it approved at the highest level possible, everyone would be in agreement with the activities that should, or should not, be performed. The job description should be reviewed periodically, and, at the least, yearly.

Records

Another frequently asked question is, *"Should I keep a record of activities during a case?"* A perfusionist, as well as every other person involved, should keep a record of activities during a case. These records may, or may not, be part of the patient's permanent medical record, depending upon the rules of the institution in which the perfusionist is practicing. The perfusionist should retain a copy of this record, either in the perfusion department, or in their own personal records, or both places.

The perfusion record should contain all information that demonstrates adherence to generally accepted standards of practice, or reasonable care. The perfusion record also should be used to document decisions or document the unusual. The record also should document lot numbers and serial numbers of equipment and devices used.

Documentation

Yet another question often asked is, *"How much is too much documentation, and how much is too little?"* The answer is really fairly simple. A perfusionist should document anything that:

1. demonstrates adherence to acceptable standards (reasonable care);
2. data that are used to make decisions or judgments; and
3. is out of the ordinary or is unusual.

A perfusionist should use the perfusion record to document adherence to generally accepted, or published standards of practice. This is in order to prove that reasonable care is practiced. By doing so, one does not avoid being sued, but one does provide, within the legal system, an opportunity for defense. Nearly all of the people involved in our legal system, especially lay people that play an important role as jurors, know very little about the practice of medicine, and even less about the practice of perfusion. They do know, however, and it is easy for an attorney to point out, when someone has not adhered to or followed generally accepted standards of practice.

In the performance of one's duties as a perfusionist, a dedicated perfusionist is required to make many decisions. It is expected of the perfusionist to make these decisions and to be able to justify them. Therefore, one should document all data that led them to make a judgment or decision. In the practice of perfusion, techniques are as variable as the number of centers that have teams performing open-heart surgery and practicing perfusion. If one is to justify the techniques they use, and the decisions they have made, they must be able to demonstrate that justification for technique and the decision-making process and judgment within the legal system. Without this documentation, it becomes extremely difficult to justify decisions.

It is equally as important to document anything that occurs during a case that is unusual or out of the ordinary. No one is expected to remember everything that occurred during any one perfusion case at some later date. Since most are filed between one and five years after the case and may not go to trial until even later, it is virtually impossible for anyone to remember all of the details, some of which may be extremely important. Given the fact that the majority of people involved in the legal system have no understanding of perfusion, it is of the utmost importance to document anything out of the ordinary. Then, at review at a later date, one may not be confronted with having to say *"I don't know," or "I can't remember."* On far too many occasions, when information is not in the record and someone does not remember, a negative influence is presented to those involved in the litigation who often have little or no understanding of the practice of perfusion.

Protocols

During the conduct of a routine perfusion case there is an indeterminate amount of details that must be attended to properly. No one should be reasonably expected to commit each and every possible detail to memory. Therefore it is encouraged, in as many areas as possible or practical, that protocols, or policies and procedures, be developed. The use of a protocol lists, organizes, details, and develops priorities for many of the intricate activities that must be performed for safe cardiopulmonary bypass. Having protocols is only part of the resolution. The important part is a strict adherence to a reasonable, practical protocol for as many different areas of responsibility as possible. Certainly the use of a prebypass checklist that includes a check of all equipment and devices being used is necessary (see Chapter 4: CHECKLISTS).

Equipment Maintenance

All permanent equipment used during a perfusion case should have periodic maintenance, and records of this maintenance should be maintained in the biomedical engineering department or perfusion department.

Instructions for Use

All manufacturers of products and devices are required to publish their recommended instructions for use with the sale of that product or device. This is a regulatory law, referred to as Good Manufacturing Practice (GMP) and is part of the device legislation passed in 1976. Any variance from these instructions must be done so at one's own risk. Any such variance from these instructions can void any warranty on the part of the seller, or manufacturer either stated or implied. If the perfusionist determines that a recommendation by a manufacturer should be ignored or modified, or that a technique described by a manufacturer should be ignored or modified, or that a piece of equipment should be used in a different way than that recommended or suggested by the manufacturer, then the perfusionist has the right to do so, and in some instances the obligation and duty to do so, but he does so at his own risk. He must be able to justify the changes or modifications to the satisfaction of the jury. Notifying the manufacturer in writing that one disagrees with the instructions for use may provide additional support for the practice if a lawsuit is filed and the perfusionist must defend the actions.

Communication

It is difficult to convey the importance of good communication during a perfusion procedure. Everyone knows, or has been told on many occasions, about the importance of communication in the operating room. An open-heart surgical team is made up of four unique and separate teams; the surgery team, the nursing team, the anesthesia team, and the perfusion team. Each team has its own important contributions to the successful outcome for a patient undergoing cardiopulmonary bypass during open-heart surgery. It is through effective communication that these four separate groups come together to create one team. Probably nowhere else, in or out of medicine, does such a situation exist that has so much importance. Each team must interact with all of the other teams effectively, with a conscious dependence on each. Effective communication, and trust among everyone involved must develop, or success will be difficult, at best. It is skilled communication that is the common thread that permits success.

AN OVERVIEW OF THE LEGAL SYSTEM

The authors of this book have had a considerable amount of experience and involvement with the legal system in the United States. No author is an attorney, but all have participated in legal cases involving perfusion, on both the plaintiff and defendant side of the case. This overview is not intended to be a legal primer, but rather an introduction to the system to provide information and familiarity for the practicing perfusionist.

Types of Law

There are three basic types of law that make up the legal system in the United States. Criminal law is written as penal codes, and it defines offenses against society as a whole. Criminal law classifies offenses as a misdemeanor or a felony, and sets punishment in terms of fines and/or imprisonment. This type of law consists of precise codes which are written by Federal, state, county, or city governments.

Common law is unwritten in statute or code, and is referred to as civil law. Judicial decisions in civil law are based on custom and precedent, and they have several sources: constitutional principles; legislation (such as the informed consent laws); judicial (precedents set by previous civil cases); and social values (such as the consumer movement). Common, or civil law is most applicable to perfusionists in the area of medical malpractice.

Regulatory law is the third basic type of law. It consists of rules and regulations written by executive enforcement agencies. These agencies include the Department of Health, the Food and Drug Administration, and the Department of Labor, among others. The rules and regulations are written so as to guide the implementation of legislative law. There is a plethora of regulatory law that affects virtually every daily activity of all working people in this country including, of course, perfusionists.

Medical Malpractice

There are four major components to medical malpractice: duty to care; breach of duty to care; injury; and proximate cause. All four components must be present in a given set of circumstances for malpractice to exist. The burden of proof in malpractice litigation is on the plaintiff.

The plaintiff must first demonstrate that a duty existed that obligated the defendant to treat the injured party. That is, it must be established that a practitioner/client relationship existed. Next the plaintiff must show that the defendant was derelict or negligent in performing the duty owed to the client. That is, it must be established that the standard of care in the particular field was not adhered to. Standard of care is defined as the degree of ability and skill maintained by other practitioners in the field in question. Thirdly, evidence must show that harm and damage befell the plaintiff.

Lastly, it must be shown that the defendant's practice and negligence was a direct proximate cause of the plaintiff's harm and damages. The "but for" test requires the plaintiff to show that the injury would not have occurred, but for the defendant's actions. The "substantial factor" test requires proof that the defendant's actions were a substantial factor in causing the damage.

ANATOMY OF A MALPRACTICE LITIGATION

First Papers

The plaintiff files a petition with the courts, naming defendants, the specific action of malpractice, the injury, and the amount of damages the plaintiff is seeking. The papers are in the form of a summons or subpoena. The named defendant should immediately notify their insurer, note when, how, and by whom the papers were served. The papers should be read carefully with an attorney, and one should be prepared to defend every item in the complaint.

Answer

The defendant's attorney must file an "answer" to the charges of the petition within a specific time period or default the action (lose the lawsuit by default). Anyone who is served with a petition must procure an attorney and file an answer to avoid default. The complaint, or petition, and answer may be amended to add charges, defendants, damages claimed, etc., after the answer is filed with the court.

After the petition and answer are filed comes the time for "discovery" for the prosecution, or plaintiff, and the time for preparing the documentation for defense. Records may by subpoenaed, and depositions may be taken from anyone that may be involved or who may be called to testify at the trial; these actions may be taken by either or both the plaintiff and defendant.

At this point a settlement may be reached out of court or the case will go forward to trial.

Settlement Out Of Court

A litigation, or lawsuit, may be settled at any time. The input of the defendant in making a settlement usually depends upon the wording of their insurance policy. An insurance policy may give the insurance company the right to negotiate and complete a settlement without the permission of the policy holder (defendant).

In a case of clear negligence, or perhaps an accident, it may be better for all parties to negotiate a settlement out of court. Paying a settlement is not an admission of guilt or negligence, though the defendant who is in the position of having no rights over the insurance carrier may well feel that the insurance carrier has pled him guilty without a trial.

ANATOMY OF A TRIAL

Choosing a Jury

A jury usually consists of twelve (12) adult men and women chosen after being questioned both by the plaintiff's attorney and the defendant's attorney.

Opening Statements

The plaintiff's attorney makes an opening statement followed by the defense attorney's opening statement. The statements consist of an outline of what each side intends to demonstrate to the jury later during the trial.

Presentation of the Plaintiff's Case

This is the point in the trial for the plaintiff to present to the court and jury all of the evidence to prove their case. The presentation may include calling the plaintiff and any other prosecution witnesses to the stand for legal testimony. The defendant has the right to cross-examine each witness. Redirect examination by the plaintiff's attorney can only cover material discussed during the cross-examination, and re-cross-examination by the defense attorney is to discuss material in the redirect examination.

Presentation of the Defense

This segment of the trial can include testimony by the defendant and other defense witnesses. All types of examination of the testimony as stated above can take place during this portion of the trial as well.

Closing Arguments

Summations of the proceedings are made by the plaintiff's attorney, followed by summation by the defense attorney, to summarize their views of the testimony.

Decision by the Jury

In some states in the United States a unanimous decision, or verdict, is required. A "hung jury" is when the jurors are unable to reach a unanimous verdict. The judge then gives instruction for further deliberation for agreement, or he may declare a mistrial at that time. If a jury continues to be unable to reach a decision a mistrial will be declared.

Damages In A Civil Suit

Awards are based on the nature of the defendant's wrongdoing rather than the result of it. Compensatory damage awards are to compensate for actual loss, and punitive damages are awarded if the defendant's behavior was deemed "willful and wanton" rather than negligent, in the action. Some states have passed laws prohibiting punitive damages in medical malpractice cases. Some states have legislated "caps" which place a ceiling on the amount of money that can be awarded in malpractice suits.

DEFINITIONS AND TERMS

Contingency Fees — payment that a plaintiff agrees to give an attorney as a specified percentage, contingent on the award paid to the plaintiff.

Deposition — sworn testimony about facts of a proceedings, or of an expert witness, given to a recorder of the court as part of the official record. Generally, both attorneys are present, and both may question the witness. Usually such testimony is taken outside the court room.

Expert Witness — a friend of the court, who provides testimony regarding a restricted area of expertise.

Product Liability — the implied warranty by the seller and/or manufacturer that the product will perform within an acceptable range if the user follows instructions.

Reasonable Care — is defined as the degree of care that a prudent practitioner would render in the same situation. This requires an expert witness to prove, or disprove.

Res Ipso Loguitor — literally means "The facts speak for themselves." This is a means of proving negligence which depends on the fact, obvious to any lay person, that the injury would not have occurred in the absence of negligence. No expert witness is required to present complex arguments or facts proving guilt.

Statute of Limitations — the time limit after the original occurrence of an incident for the filing of charges. This is a state statute and almost every state is different, varying from two to seven years. The Director of Medical Records of any hospital should be able to supply the local statutes for your information.

Vicarious Liability — when a person or institution is liable for the negligence of others (for example, employees, students, partners, etc.).

> ***"Captain of the Ship"*** doctrine states that the surgeon is in control of all employees in the operating room, and is responsible for their individual actions. In many places this doctrine is no longer in effect.
>
> ***"Responeat Superior"*** doctrine states that the employer is responsible for the negligence of employees in performance of their assigned duties, so long as the employee does not overstep the bounds of their duties.

SUMMARY

As an overview, the entire process is designed to be, and at first review appears to be, very simple and straightforward. The burden of proof is on the person making the complaint, and there is a substantial amount to be proven. However, when one adds the emotions involved with such an issue, the foreign surroundings and proceedings of a court, the potential financial losses or gains, and the total unfamiliarity of medicine to anyone involved (judge, jury, plaintiff's attorney, and even, defendant's attorney), the entire process can potentially develop into a rather life shattering crisis.

Over the last several years, we have seen very substantial awards by sympathetic or compassionate courts (depending upon one's point of view). It appears that perhaps the pendulum of time may swing the scales, back toward the middle, at least, in the near future through many of the Tort Reform measures now appearing. One thing is for certain: As long as a large portion of the public is dependent upon any small group of individuals for information, knowledge, and skills there always will be suspicion, distrust, incidents, and legal action. Such circumstances can only be exacerbated when that small group of individuals demands prime fees for such services, information, knowledge, skills, and facilities.

REFERENCES

1. Dankmyer T, Groves J: Taking steps for safety's sake. Hospitals, May 16, 60, 1977.
2. O'Connell J: Risk management for hospitals. Hospital Progress, November 40, 1974.
3. Thistle M: A look at the causes and possible solutions. Risk Management, July 10, 1977.
4. Brown B: *Risk management for hospitals.* Aspen Systems Corporation, 1979.

..LAWSUITS AND... CASENOTES

.. During cardiopulmonary bypass the surgeon inserted the left heart vent via the right superior pulmonary vein. He noted air entering the heart and removed the vent. The patient suffered severe brain damage. At deposition it was discovered that the perfusionist had inserted a cardiotomy reservoir between the vent and vent pumphead, the purpose of which was not satisfactorily explained. The perfusionist also testified that the vent worked alright once he had been notified by the surgeon and had tightened the occlusion of the vent roller head. The case settled out of court for $1,500,000.

... A staff perfusionist was operating the heart-lung machine during elective aortocoronary bypass graft surgery. During rewarming phase using wall water and a mixing valve to supply the oxygenator heat exchanger, the temperature gauge stuck without the knowledge of the perfusionist. The patient overheated and died 24 hours postoperatively. The chief perfusionist was not in the hospital at the time. The safety stop in the mixing valve was set for 37°C, but was routinely bypassed to set the water temperature at 42°C. During the inquest, the staff perfusionists testified that they had not been properly informed or given written information on how to operate the heat exchange system. The hospital paid the spouse of the deceased an undisclosed amount, and the chief perfusionist was given a suspension and demotion.

Chapter 3:

INTERFACE

Chapter 3: INTERFACE

An open-heart surgery team is not a single team, but rather a team composed of at least four separate teams. The duties and functions of a perfusionist are not performed in a vacuum, but rather as part of a team of teams, whose overall efforts are directed toward a single patient and that patient's benefit (see Chapter 1: PERFUSIONIST DUTIES AND RESPONSIBILITIES). Before the perfusionist can function well within this *team of teams*, all must be able to function as a team member within an individual team.

A single autonomous individual functioning alone has rather clear cut duties and responsibilities and a structured framework within which to function, and such an individual generally functions with a great deal of individual initiative and freedom of action. When an individual becomes a member of a team they must broaden their knowledge base and understanding not only of their actions, but also of the responsibilities and actions of other members of the team and how all team members' actions affect the actions of other team members.

Once the individual learns and accepts the team framework they will realize that they have not lost individuality or independence but rather have mastered a more complex environment in which to function, an environment in which their individual actions have a more profound impact on the outcome because of the interrelationships of the team. Thus the individual responsibilities of the team member may be viewed as having increased dramatically.

The same reasoning carried one step farther to the *team of teams* brings us to the environment in which the perfusionist functions. He is a member of the open-heart surgery team composed of the surgical team, the anesthesia team, the nursing team, and the perfusion team, none of which, in the definition of team, holds greater importance over the other for the task at hand, the surgical procedure.

However, since a team without leadership results mostly in chaos, the acknowledged team leader of the *team of teams* is the cardiothoracic surgeon. He is the individual who has brought the *team of teams* together to function for the benefit of one person, his patient.

From the team leader, the surgeon-in-charge, lines of responsibility flow naturally to the other teams. The anesthesia team, for example, is responsible for the level of consciousness of the patient, the fluid and electrolyte balance of the patient, the analgesia and amnesia of the patient, maintenance of the airway, and general homeostasis of the patient, to mention only a few functions.

The nursing team responsibilities include maintenance of sterility within the operating room, direct assistance to the surgical team in mechanical functions during the operation, anticipating the needs of the other teams, and general control of the operating room, to mention only a few functions.

The perfusion team is primarily responsible for maintenance of cardiopulmonary bypass, the fundamental function of which is maintenance of an adequate and safe level in the perfusion reservoir. Other functions include: maintenance of electrolyte and acid-base balance (see Anesthesia Team), anticipation of the needs of the operating surgeon (see Nursing Team), or maintenance of fluid balance (see Anesthesia Team). From these few examples it is obvious that the perfusion team, during the period of time involving cardiopulmonary bypass, is functioning across team responsibility lines.

The actions of the perfusion team directly affect both the nursing team and the anesthesia team, just as their actions affect the perfusion team. For example, consider the effect on perfusion when the anesthesiologist affects the acid-base balance by the administration of a vasodilator to the patient. The arterial blood pressure will fall, if elevated, and the reservoir level in the oxygenator may fall as blood volume is taken up by the patient.

Another example to consider is one in which massive blood loss occurs, the patient is hemodiluted to a hematocrit in the mid-teen range, and the perfusion flow rate and pressure are falling below acceptable levels. The patient is certainly in peril if the nursing team has not anticipated and provided for immediate blood transfusion in or near the operating room.

In both of these rather simplistic but common examples the blame is easily shifted to the anesthesia team in the first situation and the nursing team in the second. And this might be true if they were functioning independently. However, as we stated earlier, these teams do not function independently, but rather as part of the open-heart surgery team, composed of teams. The perfusionist is just as responsible, or to blame, in both cases. In the first situation, the perfusionist must know the effect of drugs added to the circuit (including the patient) during cardiopulmonary bypass and should be able to effectively communicate with the anesthesia team regarding administration of any drugs. In the second case, the perfusionist is equally charged with anticipating patient needs during open-heart surgery and should have asked if the blood had been brought up from the blood bank and had been checked.

Similarly, actions of the perfusion team can profoundly affect the other teams or operative conditions. For example, improper operation of a vent or suckers can affect the surgical field if blood is not adequately removed. Inappropriate or non-essential communication can negatively affect the surgeon's concentration during a critical phase of the procedure.

Effective communication must be established with the nursing team as well as with the anesthesia team and the surgical team. Perhaps no more harm can be done than by ineffective communication with the surgeon. There is no other procedure in medicine where the result, or outcome, is as dependent upon effective and essential communication between groups of individuals (teams) as it is in open-heart surgery.

The perfusionist can greatly increase the perfusion time by ineffective communication with the surgeon concerning suctioning, or by improper manipulation of venous drainage. The perfusionist may irreparably damage the heart by overfilling the heart and distending the left ventricle at the termination of bypass due to ineffective communication with the surgeon and/or anesthesiologist. These are but two examples of unacceptable results of ineffective communication.

Essential and effective communication during cardiopulmonary bypass involves instructions from the surgeon directed to the perfusionist or anesthesiologist, and vice versa. Acknowledgment of such instruction is mandatory, lest improper maneuvers occur because a message was misunderstood. Effective communication from the surgeon also may involve announcements regarding the status of the procedure, such as "cross-clamp is off" or "vent is out." Such announcements presage or trigger other predictable maneuvers performed by the perfusionist such as increasing flow, adding fluid to the circuit, or warming the patient according to protocol and in anticipation of weaning the patient from cardiopulmonary bypass.

Communication from the perfusionist to the surgeon involves notification that prescribed activities have been accomplished according to instruction or protocol. More importantly the surgeon is notified of any abnormal event, such as a sustained decrease in venous return or an excessively elevated arterial line pressure. The perfusionist should also communicate if a vent sucker is not functioning properly or any other observation deemed potentially threatening or of risk to the patient.

As noted earlier these communications should be acknowledged, or the communication should be repeated until the perfusionist is sure that it was heard.

Communication between anesthesiologist and perfusionist generally involves exchange of laboratory data (for example, blood gases, electrolytes, ACTs) or administration of drugs into the cardiopulmonary bypass circuit.

Communication between nursing personnel and the perfusionist generally involves confirmation that necessary perfusion supplies such as cannulae or vents and alternatives are available. Circulating nurses may also be helpful to the perfusionist by furnishing some needed manpower in a time of need or crisis. Operation of the cardiopulmonary bypass circuit and equipment is an immense responsibility, and it becomes even greater when viewed from the context of an effective team member of the open-heart surgery team, the *team of teams*.

It is mandatory that the perfusionist understand the roles of all other teams, and be able to effectively communicate with them. When this is accomplished, the perfusionist will understand that no individuality or freedom has been relinquished, but rather greater responsibility has been earned.

..LAWSUITS AND ... CASENOTES

... Four consecutive open-heart cases were performed in which the cardiotomy reservoir clotted during cardiopulmonary bypass. During investigation it was found that application of topical clotting agents at the operative site had been carried out by the surgeon without notification of the perfusionist. There were no patient injuries reported.

... The operative procedure was repair of a dissecting aneurysm of the thoracic aorta. Repair involved a graft replacement and closure of the aorta over the graft. The perfusionist noticed gross clot formation within the cardiotomy reservoir during bypass. Later it was determined that the surgeon had poured cryoprecipitate into the perigraft space prior to closure and had then sucked up the residual solution with the cardiotomy sucker. No patient injury was reported.

... At the termination of bypass the arterial pumphead was stopped and the patient was evaluated for further transfusion. When more blood was requested the perfusionist noted that blood in the oxygenator had solidified in the arterial reservoir. The patient's condition deteriorated and the patient arrested. Reinstitution of bypass was accomplished after changing and repriming the entire cardiopulmonary bypass circuit. The patient did not survive. Investigation revealed that the anesthesiologist had administered protamine to the patient without notifying the perfusionist, who had not turned off the cardiotomy suckers.

... After successful repair of a descending thoracic aneurysm the perfusionist began taking down the cardiopulmonary bypass circuit as closure of the sternum began (per Protocol). Shortly after removing the arterial line from the pumphead, the patient's arterial pressure began falling precipitously. Both surgeon and anesthesiologist diagnosed the problem simultaneously, and the arterial line was clamped. The arterial line was reinstalled in the pumphead and blood which had drained into the oxygenator through the indwelling femoral arterial cannula was transfused into the patient. The patient suffered no sequelae from the mishap.

... The surgeon clamped off the venous line without telling the perfusionist. The arterial blood reservoir was emptied and air was pumped into the patient who died on the second postoperative day.

.... The surgeon clamped off the venous line without telling the perfusionist. The arterial blood reservoir was emptied and massive air filled the arterial line, but the patient received no arterial air due to the bubble detector automatically shutting off the pump.

... The surgeon clamped off the venous line without telling the perfusionist. The arterial blood reservoir was emptied and the patient received no arterial air. The air was automatically diverted out of the arterial line through an open arterial filter purge port.

Chapter 4:

CHECKLISTS

Chapter 4: CHECKLISTS

The use of checklists in cardiopulmonary bypass is still a controversial practice. Some 77.5% of those perfusionists responding to The Survey indicated that they did use prebypass checklists of some type, but 61.2% of the time it was not written but simply "in their head" which in reality is not a checklist at all. Thus approximately 30% of the perfusionists responding utilized a written checklist. If used properly, checklists do add measurably to the safety of cardiopulmonary bypass procedures. These authors believe written checklists should be utilized on every cardiopulmonary bypass case, and they should be used properly, signed, and be made part of the patient's perfusion record.

The use of checklists probably started in aviation and was undoubtedly due to, or came about as a result of aviation accidents. However, checklists are used in other disciplines where complex technology is being employed and/or where stress, confusion, turmoil, or "business" by several people can break the concentration or train of thought of a single individual and where such a lapse could have catastrophic consequences. Space flight certainly uses extensive checklists, as do nuclear submarines, nuclear reactor power plants, intercontinental ballistic missile launch facilities, to mention only a few. It is our belief that a single open-heart surgery patient deserves no less consideration than a Boeing 747 jet aircraft full of passengers or a space shuttle with astronauts on board.

As in aviation, the checklist is most effective when used in a challenge and response manner. One perfusionist, or qualified individual, reads the checklist and the other/only perfusionist physically checks the item called out, and the first person checks the item off on the checklist. When completed, both individuals should sign the checklist and keep it with the perfusion record. As a legal document for the perfusionist's defense, it will have much more credibility if completed by two persons and signed by those persons.

If only one perfusionist is available in an open-heart program, they should train someone, for example a circulating nurse or scrub technician, to assist them with the checklist and require them to sign the checklist upon completion.

It is certainly acceptable that one person utilize a checklist, and this situation is preferable to no checklist at all, but it simply does not have the credibility as one completed by two people. It is all too easy for the plaintiff's attorney to imply or state that the single perfusionist simply checked off the boxes and did not really use the checklist properly. Then it is the perfusionist's word against that of the attorney across the body of the dead or injured patient.

One additional item should be included which properly goes on the checklist, but which practically belongs on the perfusion flow chart (see Figure 5.3). Since most low level alarm sensors and bubble detectors work on principles which involve blood and since most perfusion circuits are primed with clear crystalloid solutions, these alarm devices cannot be turned on prior to commencing cardiopulmonary bypass. When the start of bypass is not routine and is hurried, as in the case of a failed PTCA where the patient may well be receiving cardiopulmonary resuscitation, turning on the alarms may be easily overlooked in the priorities of the moment and may not be included in the perfusionist's train of thought. With the **ALARMS ON** appearing on the perfusion record, the perfusionist is reminded of this item the first time they make a chart entry (see Chapter 5: CHARTING).

Checking the mechanical function and electrical and electronic components of the heart-lung machine will only tell the perfusionist that they were functional at the time they were turned on and were checked, but nothing more. Such checks will not ensure that the machine will function properly the next time it is turned on. Likewise, preventive maintenance inspections will not guarantee that the machine will function properly five minutes after the maintenance technician leaves the operating room. However, such checks and inspections are mandatory in that they may uncover some potentially hazardous existing condition. But the perfusionist must not be lulled into a false sense of security and must always be alert to machine failure and must have thought ahead and planned ahead for such an eventuality.

The first things that should appear on the checklist should be the mechanical, electrical, and electronic systems. This includes not only the heart-lung machine but also the heat exchange system, monitoring system, and any other apparatus utilized during cardiopulmonary bypass. Also included in this section should be the presence of emergency handcranks and spare fuses. This section could appear under the heading of **HARDWARE.**

The next section should be the **DISPOSABLE COMPONENTS** of the system, and it should begin with sterile integrity and the proper type and size devices for the particular patient.

The next section could be **ASSEMBLY** and would include whether the tubing is placed through the pumps in the proper direction, the lines are clear and free, connected properly to the oxygenator, cardiotomy reservoir, filters, etc. **GAS SYSTEM** should be in this section or in a separate section at this point in the checklist and should include function of the flow meters and/or blender, integrity of gas lines and the correct type of gas source, gas filters, etc.

The next section should be **PHARMACOLOGY** and should include sterility of the priming solution, correct type of priming solution, and expiration date, etc. The same should be included in checking any drugs added by the perfusionist to the priming solution or to any drugs drawn up by the perfusionist and kept on the pump. The pump should be primed and debubbled at this point.

The next section could be **SYSTEM CHECK** and would begin with inspection for bubbles, recirculating and setting occlusions, checking suction and vent for the proper flow direction, and checking for the performance of both devices, setting any computers or monitors with proper patient data such as patient weight, BSA, etc.

The **FINAL CHECKLIST** could include function checks of the alarms, presence of any needed ancillary equipment, emergency spares of whatever, water source, hypothermia source, etc. The time and initial dose of heparin administered may also be on this checklist.

Because of the vast variation in cardiopulmonary bypass systems and types of hardware used, no complete checklist has been supplied for the reader. The authors have provided a skeleton of a checklist which the individual perfusionist or perfusion team can flesh out and modify to fit their particular needs. The authors caution that there is no known substitute for the perfusionist's brain, knowledge, experience, and prior planning for emergencies. The checklist is a useful adjunct and nothing more. It is not sacrosanct or chiseled in granite nor static or unchanging. If the perfusion checklist does not include all pertinent items which could lead to a set of circumstances that result in perfusion misadventure, the perfusionist certainly could be lulled into a false sense of security or in fact led down a path to disaster; a path which he himself charted and mapped.

The authors believe that checklists should be used, should be used properly and should be used in the proper perspective. The checklist is not an excuse not to think.

..LAWSUITS AND ...CASE NOTES

.. During cardiopulmonary bypass for aortocoronary bypass graft surgery the perfusionist allowed the arterial reservoir of the oxygenator to empty. An unknown amount of air was pumped into the patient and the anesthesiologist was the first to alert the team after hearing a strange noise which was air rushing through the coronary grafts which had been anastomosed distally. The patient never regained consciousness and was disconnected from life support on the second postoperative day and died immediately. Plaintiff filed suit against the surgeon, hospital, perfusionist and anesthesiologist. During deposition it was established that no checklist was used by the perfusionist and that the perfusionist had never turned on the low level alarm sensor or the bubble detector. The case was settled out of court for an amount in excess of $800,000.

... During routine cardiopulmonary bypass the perfusionist noted a deterioration in consecutive blood gas results. Increasing the gas-to-blood flow ratio did not appreciably affect the problem. Inspection of the entire system revealed a cracked gas filter which was leaking gas into the room. The perfusionist did not use a checklist. The patient suffered no detectable injury.

... During administration of cold blood cardioplegia at 4°C an increased resistance was noted in the cardioplegia line. Cardioplegia was infused one time. When the coronary vessel was opened the surgeon discovered gross clot formation. Further examination of the coronary vasculature revealed clot through out the system. The patient was pronounced dead on the operating table. The perfusionist was not using a checklist. No one observed the positive cold agglutinin report.

... During routine cardiopulmonary bypass the oxygenator failed to oxygenate. While inspecting the entire system the perfusionist discovered a clamp on the gas line. The pump had been set up by a perfusion assistant. The primary perfusionist was not using a checklist. The operation continued uneventfully.

Chapter 5:

CHARTING

Chapter 5: CHARTING

The primary purpose of charting for the perfusionist is to create a permanent record of the events that occurred during the conduct of cardiopulmonary bypass. If performed properly, charting serves another extremely useful purpose, that of prompting the perfusionist to observe and perform as well as record relevant acts, facts, and happenings. It is all too easy, during a long and uneventful aortocoronary bypass graft procedure, for example, to become unmindful of the seemingly more minor aspects of the bypass. If charting is properly performed, the perfusionist is reminded to perform or note these aspects. A chart might well be thought of as an ongoing checklist for cardiopulmonary bypass. With a properly utilized chart the perfusionist should be able to reconstruct the entire cardiopulmonary bypass procedure days, weeks, or even years after the occurrence of the procedure.

In today's world of perfusion the chart that adequately suffices is often two pages in length. There does not seem to be a chart capable of holding all relevant information which is comprised of only one page. However, two pages seems a bit much. Alternatively, the prebypass checklist (see Chapter 4: CHECKLISTS) can be part of the two-page chart. There is no valid reason why the prebypass checklist cannot be part of the patient's chart, and there are many valid reasons why it should be.

The original copy of cardiopulmonary bypass chart or record should be part of the patient's hospital record and in hospitals where this is not the case, the perfusionist would be well advised to insist that this medical record procedure be established. A carbon copy should be retained by the perfusion department or office. In hospitals where one does not exist, for example in some contract perfusion situations, the perfusionist should retain a carbon copy of the record permanently in his/her personal files; actually this is not a bad idea for all perfusionists to follow.

Malpractice suits have variable statutes of limitation depending upon the particular state. Five or six years after the procedure is not the time to start trying to locate a copy of the perfusion record or to create a satisfactory record in the first place. Thus the perfusionist should retain the first copy and ensure that it is legible. Charting should be done in ink, preferably a fine point ball point pen, and in the case of multiple copies, with a heavy hand.

If errors are made on the chart the changes should be initialed and both the error and the correct information should be clearly legible. The preferred method is to draw a thin line through the mistake in such a way that it is still readable and then to write the correct information immediately above, below or to the side of the error and initialing your correction. Erasures or write-overs are very difficult to satisfactorily explain to a jury.

Some interest has been generated from time to time in the actual type or structure of the perfusion record, usually by the anesthesiology department. The interest takes the direction of changing the common and accepted columnar time and data format, Figure 5.1, to the flow chart type usually utilized by anesthesiologist. This type of chart is very useful to the anesthesiologist, but it must be remembered that they have used this type of charting from the very first day of their training and are very familiar with its use. Changing the perfusion record world wide would be very difficult and prove very confusing for some time to come. It is not at all clear that this type of format is really adaptable to the information which should be charted by the perfusionist. A combination chart which includes a flow type section is shown in Figure 5.2.

The record should be stamped with the patient's hospital name plate, and the perfusionist should record all pertinent data prior to bypass. Alternatively, this information including patient's name, hospital identification number, age, and gender, may be written on the perfusion record. The pertinent data should include: date, weight, height, Body Surface Area (if utilized), diagnosis, scheduled procedure, surgeon(s), anesthesiologist, allergies, blood type, preexisting pathological conditions such as diabetes, AIDS, hepatitis, syphilis, whether the patient has had previous cardiac surgery, etc., initial heparin dose and time given, most recent Hgb and Hct, or include this information from the prebypass blood gas analysis. A prebypass blood gas analysis should be performed shortly prior to the beginning of cardiopulmonary bypass, at that time the patient's blood pressure and temperature should also be recorded. Notation of priming volume and desired blood flow rate should be recorded. In multiple surgeon centers or for contract perfusionists operating in several

SURGEON: ______ DATE: ______ CASE NO: ______

WEIGHT: ______ LB ______ Kg.

PARTIAL BYPASS: ON: ______ OFF: ______ TOTAL TIME: ______

COMPLETE BYPASS: ON: ______ OFF: ______ Complete Time: ______

ISCHEMIC TIME ______

FLOW RATE: ______ CC/Kg./MIN. ______ CC/MIN.

PRIME: ______ ______ ML
______ ______ ML

ADDED: ______ ML | TOTAL ______ ML

EBL: ______ ML | BAGGED ______ ML

URIN: ______ ML | RETURNED ______ ML

	TIME	FLOW	BP	TEMP.	Hgb	O_2/CO_2	pH	pCO_2	pO_2	Na	K	COMMENTS
						/						
						/						
						/						
						/						
						/						
						/						
						/						
						/						
						/						
						/						
						/						
						/						
						/						
						/						
						/						
						/						
						/						
						/						
						/						
						/						

DIAGNOSIS:

OXYGENATOR ______
CARDIOTOMY ______
FILTER ______
TUBING ______
ROOM BYPASS URINE

PROCEDURE:

CARDIOPULMONARY BYPASS

0-88 8/87

PATIENT CHART

Figure 5.1 A sample of perfusion record of the time and entry type.

Date ____
Pump No. ____
☐ Elective ☐ Urgent ☐ Emergency
Diagnosis ____
Procedure ____
Surgeons ____
Perfusionists ____
Anesthesiologists ____

Equipment
Pump ____
Oxygenator ____
CDS Res. ____
KAS Res. ____
Heat Exch. ____
Filters ____
Tubing ____
Other ____

Height ____ cm
Weight ____ kg
BSA ____ m^2
Flow ____ ml/min
@ ____ $L/m^2/min$

Blood Type ____
Allergies ____

Cannulation	Arterial	Venous
Site		
Catheter		
Line		

Fluids	Urine Output	Blood Loss	Replace	BALANCE
Pre				
During				

Perfusate
Crystalloid ____ ml
Blood ____ cc
Colloid ____ cc
Other ____ ml
____ ml
Prime Total ____ ml

Total Pump Fluids
____ ml
____ cc
____ cc
____ ml
____ ml
Total ____ ml

HEPARIN
Amt. ____ mg
Time ____

Aortic Cross Clamp Time
ON ____ +
OFF ____ +
TOTAL ____

Pre-op Coagulopathy ☐ Yes ☐ No
Halothane/Ethrane ☐ Yes ☐ No
Cardiovascular Drugs ☐ Yes ☐ No
Pre Pump ☐ 1
During ☐ 2
Post Pump ☐ 3

Prime Additives ____

Bypass Time

ON	Partial	Total	OFF	Total	Partial	TOTAL

O_2 G:B / % O_2
pH
pCO_2
pO_2
AO_2%
B.E.
VpO_2
VO_2%
Hgb
Hct
K
Na
Glu

ACT
Pre Pump ____
Post Heparin ____
Post Pump ____

120, 110, 100, 90, 80, 70, 60, 50, 40, 30, 20, 10
Anes. % 1.0, .5, 0
Minutes 20 40 60 80 100 120 140 160 180 200
TEMP. ☐ R ☐ B(●) ☐ NP
38°C 36°C 34°C 32°C 30°C 28°C 26°C 24°C 22°C 20°C 18°C

(X) MEAN ARTERIAL PRESSURE mm/Hg (→) CARDIAC INDEX (−) FLOW ml/min

Disposition Perfusate
Reinfused: ____ cc
To Anesthesiologist ____ cc
Disposed ____ cc
Ultrafiltration ____ ml

NOTES:

Card Suction L M H

Prepared by ____

Myocardial Protection K = mEq
Est. CPS ____ ml

	Vol	Temp	Time	Site
Initial	ml	°C	+	
Other	ml	°C	+	
	ml	°C	+	
	ml	°C	+	
	ml	°C	+	
	ml	°C	+	

Total CPS ____ ml Countershock ☐ Yes ☐ No

Form 2208 Rev. 6/87

Figure 5.2 A sample of a perfusion record of the combination flow type and the time and entry type.

hospitals, identification of the primary surgeon and the anesthesiologist should be made on the chart. Other pertinent information that should be recorded includes: variation from protocol of site of arterial and venous cannulation, size of cannulae and arterial and venous lines.

Every single piece of disposable equipment should be listed by manufacturer or model number including an identification number, such as serial number, lot number, etc. This is of vital importance to the perfusionist. In centers where more than one heart-lung machine is routinely utilized a notation of which machine was used on the case should be made.

The record should begin with the commencement of bypass. The time should be noted as well as any abnormal events such as, "emergency from cath lab-CPR in progress," "emergency-failed PTCA," "emergency from ICU-CPR in progress," "emergency from Elsewhere General Hospital," or simply "emergency." There should be some reminder to the perfusionist that this was not a normal scheduled case. Initial blood and gas flow rates, blood pressure, and the patient's temperature should be recorded. It is also advisable to provide a space to record the turning on of the bubble detector, low level alarm sensor, or other safety devices (see Figure 5.3). If a blender is used, and only with a membrane oxygenator and with an oxygen sensor inline downline, the oxygen percent should be noted as well as either actual gas flow rate or gas-to-blood flow ratio.

During bypass an entry should be made every time a change is made by the perfusionist in any of the perfusion controls or parameters or anytime one of the monitored values changes. During an absolutely stable perfusion an entry should be made at least every 15 minutes. When an entry is made it is very important that all the blanks for that line be filled in beginning with the time. Military or 24 hour time is a useful tool in today's world of around the clock open-heart surgery in that it automatically differentiates AM from PM. Blood gas values should be recorded on the chart at the time the sample is drawn and not when the results are received. Blood gas samples should be drawn shortly after changing either the gas or blood flow rate or changing the temperature of the arterial blood or the patient's temperature (see Chapter 12: CONDUCT OF PERFUSION).

Each and every time during bypass the perfusionist is directed to deviate from the perfusion protocol a chart entry should be made which includes who directed the action such as, "level lowered/anest," "flow reduced/surg," or "pump stopped/surg." Cardiopulmonary bypass is a prescription situation and noting who directed the action is the perfusionist's authorization to deviate from protocol. It is extremely important that the perfusionist be able to explain to the satisfaction of a jury why they deviated from what was normally done during cardiopulmonary bypass or what would be the national or accepted standard of practice or action during bypass in a similar situation.

	TIME	FLOW	BP	TEMP.	Hgb	O_2/CO_2	pH	pCO_2	pO_2	Na	K	COMMENTS
PRE:		X				/						
ON:						/						
		X	X	X	X	X / X	X	X	X	X	X	:ALARMS ON:
						/						
						/						
						/						
						/						

Figure 5.3 Shows a section of a perfusion record which has pre-printed entries for PREbypass blood gas results, ON bypass notation, and ALARMS ON notation. Note all non-applicable blanks are filled in with Xs in keeping with the policy of filling in each blank in the line at each time notation.

All fluids added to the bypass circuit should be recorded at the time they are added and identified as to composition and volume or dose such as "500cc D5RL," "1 unit PRC," etc. Any and all drugs added by the perfusionist to the bypass circuit should be charted as well as the authority for such addition such as "300 mg heparin/anest," "1 amp Sodium Bicarb./prot.," etc. Perfusionists are not permitted by law to blithely give prescription, or other, medications to patients either directly or through the bypass circuit. They are not permitted by law to prescribe such medications either. Perfusionists may administer medications on or by prescription of a qualified licensed physician, and such prescription may be verbal or in the form of either a written or verbal order; a perfusion protocol constitutes such an order. However, just as a Registered Nurse must be able to show authorization for administration of medications, so must the perfusionist. It is much easier to establish the daily use of this written or verbal protocol on an ongoing basis rather than have to try to explain why it was not done on every case. Thus it is mandatory that the perfusionist record both medication and authority of every drug they add to the perfusion circuit, even intravenous fluid therapy which is a prescription medication.

Because of the vital importance of adequate anticoagulation during cardiopulmonary bypass, activated clotting time (ACT) results should be noted on the perfusion record, or alternatively, on the anesthesia record. Additionally, if an ultrafiltration device is used during bypass, the time of use and volumes of plasma water (ultrafiltrate) removed should be noted. If cardioplegia solution is administered by the perfusionist, the time and volumes given should be recorded. Myocardial temperature may also be recorded if measured.

Termination of cardiopulmonary bypass should be recorded. Although not commonly done, it is a good idea to record one or two sets of patient hemodynamic monitoring values after termination of bypass. Inclusion of such information indicates how the patient was doing at 10 or 20 minutes postbypass. Both the volume and disposition of all fluid remaining in the cardiopulmonary bypass circuit should be recorded, such as, "300 cc transfused, 500 cc to ICU with pt.", "750 cc to blood bank;" what happened to it after that is not usually the responsibility of the perfusionist. If a cell washer is used by the perfusionist, the volume of blood and hematocrit of such blood returned to the patient should be noted. If a hemoconcentrator was employed, the volume of fluid extracted should be recorded.

If an accident should occur during bypass it must be noted. There are preferable ways to record such occurrences. It is unwise to record, for example, "massive air pumped into the patient." Instead, a notation of "pump stopped to clear arterial line" tells the same story as does "arterial reservoir level lost" or "arterial reservoir level below minimum." "Reversed sump or vent" also tells a complete story. The results are usually available in ICU for anyone to see, at least for a few days. To ignore or to attempt to cover up such a happening is unethical, and in today's world just will not work.

Finally, the surgical procedure actually performed should be recorded being specific, such as, "CAB X2 or 3," "AVR-St.Jude," "MVR REDO-Bjork," etc. Model number, size, and serial number of the implanted prosthesis may be recorded for the surgeon's convenience.

Once the chart has been reviewed for completeness and legibility it should be at least initialed. Some perfusionists prefer to "sign off" the case, but the purpose for such a notation is to be able to identify the perfusionist who actually did the case. There are some exceptional operating room settings where no identification is preferable, but they are rare.

..LAWSUITS AND ...CASE NOTES

.. Patient with a documented history of hypertension and syncope suffered neurological damage during aortocoronary bypass graft surgery. Review of the perfusion record revealed that the first blood gas results drawn nine minutes after the start of bypass indicated an arterial pO_2 of 65 mmHg and a perfusion pressure of 44 mmHg. The next blood gas sample was drawn 41 minutes later with no corrections noted in the gas flow rate and the blood flow rate reduced by 10% in the interim. The perfusion pressure rose gradually to 78 mmHg during this period. A malpractice suit was filed against the surgeon and perfusionist. The case settled out of court for an amount in excess of $475,000.

.. Patient suffered neurological damage during aortocoronary bypass graft surgery. Five years later, at deposition, the perfusion record could not be located by either the hospital or the chief perfusionist, who testified at deposition that they recalled doing the case. The perfusion record was not a part of the patient's hospital record at the time, or in fact, five years later. A malpractice suit was filed alleging an air embolic event during cardiopulmonary bypass. An arterial filter was used during the case but the vent line was closed. This case settled out of court in excess of $150,000.

.. Patient suffered neurological damage during repair of congenital heart defect. Four years later the perfusion team could not identify who was the primary perfusionist during the case and consequently could not identify a person to defend the perfusion record at deposition. This case was dismissed due to a technical error committed by plaintiff's attorney. Ultimately the plaintiff filed a malpractice suit against their former attorney.

.. Patient suffered minimal or questionable brain damage during aortocoronary bypass graft surgery. A malpractice suit was filed against everyone in sight and every equipment manufacturer. The perfusion record was negative but hospital records indicated an arterial blood gas sample on bypass which was definitely unsatisfactory as far as the pO_2 value was concerned. This value had been written over and a normal value was written in. No one could be found who could explain either who made the change or why the change was made. Case settled out of court, award unknown.

.. Patient suffered severe brain damage during cardiopulmonary bypass for repair of a congenital heart defect. Perfusion record revealed an extremely long period of partial bypass and hypotension. The records also indicated a great variance between two arterial blood samples drawn from the aortic root and from the oxygenator with no indication that the perfusionist had made any attempt to correct the discrepancy and no indication that the perfusionist had either attempted to increase the flow rate or perfusion pressure or had informed anyone of the long period of hypoperfusion and hypotension. The anesthesia record was also mute on these subjects. A malpractice suit was filed against the hospital, the perfusionist, the surgeon, and the anesthesiologist.

Chapter 6:

BLOOD AND BLOOD HANDLING

Chapter 6: BLOOD AND BLOOD HANDLING

The authors will not go into the descriptive anatomy of this vital tissue, but refer the reader to innumerable specialized texts on the subject. Likewise, the references for HIV (AIDS) are so numerous and are being updated monthly so that to list them may well be meaningless.

In the early days of open-heart surgery and cardiopulmonary bypass the oxygenating devices that were used required large priming volumes and consequently large volumes of blood. Some open-heart programs plateaued numerically due to the limitations of the hospital blood bank or even the community. Pediatric surgery in the early years required fresh heparinized blood which had to be collected, typed and cross-matched within 24 hours of surgery and use.

It was this problem that gave birth to the crystalloid prime, hemodilution perfusion, and its rapid acceptance in the open-heart operating room. As blood banks and communities geared up physically and psychologically to the wonders and needs of open-heart surgery, the use of hemodilution tended to slip from its pure state into one of hemodilution plus blood plus an assortment of other additives to the perfusion circuit.

It was the sudden appearance of and rapid spread of hepatitis that brought hemodilution back to a pure state. Blood banks became very adept at screening for the hepatitis virus and the practice of hemodilution perfusion slipped once again. During this period, for reasons unknown to these authors, the perioperative and subsequent postoperative treatment of the open-heart patient included large volumes of fresh frozen plasma. [As a point of information, from one unit of blood the recipient stands the risk of contracting a disease from only one person, the donor. From a unit of fresh frozen plasma, the patient stands the risk of contracting a disease from 15 people since a unit of fresh frozen plasma is the result of 15 pooled units.]

AIDS

Due to this indiscriminate use of fresh frozen plasma, some open-heart programs experienced a return of the white lung syndrome, also called the pump lung or shock lung syndrome, and a very few experienced cases of AIDS retrospectively in their open-heart patients. At the same time the HIV virus was identified and AIDS patients began appearing across the United States. The attendant horror of the disease and the fear of the community, and particularly the health care worker who was constantly exposed to the body fluids of untested patients, became reality. With these factors looming large over the operating theater hemodilution has experienced a return to the pure state, as well it should.

The risk factor of contracting AIDS for the perfusionist is the highest of any of the allied health care professionals and equal to that of the operating surgeon, the surgical assistant and the scrub nurse. The Survey data has shown that 4.6% of perfusionists had contracted blood-borne diseases in the course of operating cardiopulmonary bypass equipment. The inevitability of a perfusionist contracting AIDS sometime in the future and on the job is apparent to these authors. It may even be that perfusionists are already victims and in the incubation stage at this time. For these and other obvious reasons, the perfusionist must strictly adhere to the guidelines which have been developed in an effort to protect them, their families and close friends, and other health care workers from contracting this currently universally lethal disease.

The perfusionist must:

1. Wear at all times in the operating room scrub clothes plus **disposable** mask, cap,

gloves, gown which is fluid-proof and full sleeved, and glasses or goggles of the type that prevents fluid splash entry from the side of the eye. Perfusionists who wear glasses or contacts can obtain goggles which will fit over the glasses and which provide protection from the side as well.

2. Be particularly vigilant in handling "sharps:" needles, syringes, surgical blades, and scissors. More manipulation is done with "sharps" than one might first imagine, considering ACTs, drawing blood gas samples, cutting tubing and nicking a glove, thus breaching the protection the gloves offer. "Sharps" must be disposed of in a puncture-proof container such as a glass IV solution bottle immediately after use. They should not be allowed to remain on the pump or utility cart until a later more convenient time. Needles should not be recapped, and extreme care should be used when injecting with a needle such as when performing an ACT test where blood must be transferred to a test tube.
3. Blood spills or contamination should be cleaned up promptly, **"sharps" should not be cleaned**, with a solution of 5.25% sodium hypochlorite diluted 1:10. Household bleach is 5.25% sodium hypochlorite. Once prepared, the solution should not be saved over night. If in doubt, clean it with the sodium hypochlorite solution. With AIDS it is better to be safe than regretful.
4. The same precautions should be observed when working with patients outside the operating room in special situations, particularly during procedures such as ECMO, LVAD, IABP or emergency cardiopulmonary bypass support.
5. Until such time as general patient screening for AIDS is in force, the perfusionist would be well advised to wear protective clothing, gloves, mask, and goggles in any patient contact situation and to consider that each patient is HIV positive.
6. Any injury, wounds or puncture injuries should be reported to the appropriate hospital authority, and a hospital accident/incident report should be completed. The perfusionist should keep a copy of this report in a safe place. Emergency Room or other proper medical treatment should be obtained immediately. In The Survey 35% of the perfusionists responding indicated that they had been injured while operating the heart-lung machine during cardiopulmonary bypass.
7. After cardiopulmonary bypass the entire circuit including oxygenator and reservoir must be disposed of in a safe fashion. The components and all residual fluid should be carefully placed in a water-proof container and sealed. Disposal should be with the other operating room debris.

BLOOD TRANSFUSION

The procedure of human blood transfusion is a prescription procedure authorized only on and by order of a physician, and administered only by approved, trained personnel. This prescription may be by direct verbal order, written order, or written protocol. It is not in the purview of the perfusionist to diagnose the need for a blood transfusion or to order a blood transfusion under any circumstances. The perfusionist's involvement in blood transfusion should be limited to the addition of properly checked blood to the cardiopulmonary bypass circuit on order, after appropriate training in such administration.

The perfusionist should not be one of those persons checking the blood to be administered. The perfusionist does not have the training and should not accept the responsibility of checking blood donor units. Consider the situation in which transfusion is to occur during cardiopulmonary bypass: who is watching the bypass circuit, specifically the arterial blood reservoir level, while the perfusionist is checking blood slip numbers against blood bag numbers? Hospitals have written protocols that address the process of blood administration, and most have separate protocols for the operating room. The perfusionist is not included in these protocols and should not be. Perfusionists responding to The Survey indicated that 25% had observed a life-threatening transfusion reaction within the last three years with 33 deaths and 5 permanent injuries.

Once a properly checked unit of blood has been handed to the perfusionist, they should ask who checked the unit and should not administer it until they receive two identifying answers. Once this has been established, the perfusionist should reconstitute the units of blood following formal protocols. When this has been done the blood should be added to the perfusion circuit. Bagged blood should not be left lying on the heart-lung machine. Human blood belongs either in the circulating fluid of the bypass circuit or in the blood storage refrigerator. Human blood has a limited safe time that it can remain at room temperature before deleterious changes begin to occur.

A common method of reconstituting human blood is:

Adding 2000 units of heparin to the unit of blood, (1000 units for packed red cells) and adding one milliequivalent of sodium bicarbonate per 100ml of total prime. 0.4 grams of calcium chloride is added to the circulating prime. There is absolutely no reason to add calcium chloride to the unit of blood and at least one good reason not to add it to the unit of blood, namely the possibility of coagulation occurring due to poor mixing of the heparin.

These guidelines are given only as an example and any well considered protocol for reconstituting would suffice (see Chapter 14: PEDIATRIC CONSIDERATIONS).

Addition of the blood to the bypass circuit should be done with filtration either by passage through a transfusion filter or by adding the blood to the inlet side of a filtered cardiotomy reservoir or to a cardiotomy reservoir which has an extracorporeal filter between the cardiotomy reservoir and the oxygenator.

HEMOLYSIS

Hemolysis is the destruction or dissolution of the formed elements of the blood, red cells, white cells, and platelets. It is customarily thought of as mechanical destruction of red cells with the accompanying increase in free plasma hemoglobin leaked from the injured or destroyed red cell membrane. Normal free plasma hemoglobin production during cardiopulmonary bypass is in the range of 25-35 mg% per hour, but is not linear beyond 120-150 minutes. With longer perfusion time the hemolysis rate generally increases dramatically.

The second part of the word hemolysis is *lysis*, the dissolution of cells. This destruction of cells is due not only to the mechanical considerations of blood damaged in the cardiopulmonary bypass circuit, but to the action of chemical substances produced by the body, to the action of chemical substances released by the injured cells, and to the action of chemical substances not naturally occurring in the body but produced during the process of cardiopulmonary bypass. It is this aspect of hemolysis that is the most insidious.

Autotransfusion produces many of these non-naturally occurring substances and, if not washed off before reinfusion, can destroy healthy cells within the body. This is probably the cause of the early adverse reports in the use of autotransfusion.[1-3] The use of suction systems can produce the same results. Greater than 90% of the hemolysis occurring during cardiopulmonary bypass occurs in the suction system.[4-6] It is important that the suction system be used properly during cardiopulmonary bypass in order to reduce hemolysis and minimize the potential side effects (see Chapter 12: CONDUCT OF PERFUSION).

The entire perfusion circuit also plays a part in hemolysis during cardiopulmonary bypass. State-of-the-art manufacturing has minimized rough surfaces, parting lines, bumps, spurs and ridges on the components of the extracorporeal circuit. The one factor that has not changed is the hemolysis occurring when blood flows across different types of material. Adjacent dissimilar materials cause a change in electrical charge when blood flows across the junction and hemolysis occurs. The perfusionist can minimize this effect by keeping the changes in material to a minimum.

There is some validity to the thought that silicone rubber tubing used in the pumphead section of the suction and vent lines will reduce mechanical hemolysis.

REFERENCES

1. Reed CC, Milam JD, Sabawala PB, Wukasch DC, Cooley DA: Autotransfusion new or used? JECT 5:42, 1973.
2. Watson CM, Watson JR: Autotransfusion: Review of American literature with report of two additional cases. Am J Surg 33:232,1974.
3. Rakower SR, Worth MH: Autotransfusion: Perspective and critical problems. J Trauma 13:573, 1973.
4. Keenan RM, Keen WR, Taylor DE, Crane TN, Reed CC: A comparative hemolysis study of bubble oxygenators. AmSECT Proceed 2:39, 1974.
5. Keen WR, Reed CC: Iatrogenic hemolysis: A critical study. AmSECT Proceed 3:22, 1975.
6. Clark DK, Reed CC, Keen WE, Crane TN: Pericardial hemolysis: A critical study. AmSECT Proceed 4:57, 1976.

..LAWSUITS AND ... CASE NOTES

.. During bypass the primary perfusionist was handed two units of blood to add to the perfusion circuit by the second perfusionist. Allegedly the blood had been checked by the circulating nurse and the second perfusionist. The primary perfusionist did not ask. A few minutes later the circulating nurse realized that the patient had been given another intended recipient's blood. The operation was completed and the patient underwent two complete blood exchanges while on bypass. The patient developed generalized DIC in the recovery room and died on the second postoperative day. A lawsuit was filed against the primary perfusionist, the hospital, and the surgeons. It was settled out of court for an amount in excess of $1,000,000.

...The patient was undergoing surgical repair of a ventricular septal defect. Bypass was begun without the perfusionist asking the anesthesiologist if the heparin had been given. The anesthesiologist was responsible for this activity with this particular open-heart team. Bypass proceeded for 27 minutes before the anesthesiologist realized that the heparin was still in the syringe on his cart. Heparin was given and bypass was terminated 15 minutes later. The patient suffered no observable ill effects. The priming solution in this institution contained 2500 units of heparin per liter of crystalloid solution. It is believed that this small amount of heparin offered enough protection in this instance to avert disaster. It well may be that the patient was also experiencing sub-clinical DIC which was reversed with the addition of the proper heparin dosage.

..The patient, an R.N., was undergoing cardiopulmonary bypass for surgical correction of a congenital heart defect. The units of blood had been checked by the second perfusionist and the director of the operating room, an R. N. The units were checked outside the operating room and then given to the primary perfusionist who was operating the cardiopulmonary bypass circuit. The blood was added to the bypass circuit and then it was discovered that the blood administered was of the wrong blood type and the recipient was the wrong sex.

Surgery was completed and the patient transferred to ICU. The patient suffered a complete renal shutdown and was hemodialyzed repeatedly. At the end of the second month of hospitalization the accounting office of the hospital sent the patient's family a bill for hospital care to date and strongly urged immediate payment. The patient's brother, an attorney, apparently took exception to this sort of treatment and suit was filed against the hospital and all involved. The patient was discharged on the 127th postoperative day.

The case was settled out of court for an amount equal to all hospital bills plus $1,000,000.

...The cardiopulmonary bypass circuit was assembled and primed using the routine protocol which included the addition of blood to the perfusate. The blood was handed to the perfusionist who neither asked nor was informed that the blood unit had been checked. Just prior to starting bypass the circulating nurse discovered that the blood added to the bypass circuit was intended for transfusion to another patient. The complete bypass circuit was discarded along with the priming fluid, and a new set-up was used on the patient who suffered no ill effects.

... During reconstitution of a unit of blood the perfusionist was adding heparin to the blood bag. The perfusionist inserted the needle into the blood bag outlet, through the side of the unit of blood and into his hand. He did not report the injury to either his supervisor or the hospital nor did he fill out an incident report or go to the emergency room for treatment When he developed hepatitis several weeks later the hospital took the position that it was not job related and he received only minimal benefits while convalescing. Upon recovery he found another perfusion job.

... During attempted administration of cold blood cardioplegia it was observed that the infusion pressure was increasing alarmingly. Administration was stopped and clot was discovered in the cardioplegia system line. Investigation postoperatively revealed that an unreported cold agglutinin was present in the patient. The patient's recovery was uneventful.

Chapter 7:

TUBING AND CIRCUITS

Chapter 7: TUBING AND CIRCUITS

TUBING

The tubing most commonly used in cardiopulmonary bypass today is polyvinyl chloride (PVC). Some limited usage of silicone rubber tubing in the roller pumphead is found in the older programs. Other compounds have been evaluated through the years but have proven to be either impractical, unsuitable, or too expensive.

Polyurethane at one time was thought to be the perfect tubing but was excessively expensive. It is more biocompatable, tougher and longer wearing, less susceptible to spallation, but is of a higher durometer, or harder, than PVC. One manufacturer seemed to be on the right track with a co-extruded tubing which was full thickness PVC on the outside with a liner of polyurethane tubing on the inside. Unfortunately, the two dissimilar tubings often separated during use in the roller pumphead or when the perfusionist inserted a connector in the tubing, and the project was abandoned.

PVC tubing is manufactured by extrusion of solid, very hard polyvinyl chloride pellets into PVC tubing using high pressure and heat. The high pressure itself creates additional heat which, during manufacture, is only partially dissipated prior to coiling and storage of the tubing. Not completely cooling the tubing prior to coiling is the first step in "setting" the tubing. Subsequent manufacture into tubing packs utilizes ethylene oxide sterilization processing which in itself has a heating component in the sterilization cycle and adds further to "setting" a curve into the tubing. PVC tubing has another component called memory which is the ability of the tubing to return to its previous shape once it has been deformed in some manner, such as being compressed by the roller head of the pump. This memory in the PVC tends to return a straightened piece of PVC to the curved shape that has been "set" into it by both the extrusion and tubing pack manufacturing process.

The perfusionist should not fight this curvature, but rather let the curved PVC work for him. The natural curve of the tubing fits nicely into the backing plate of the roller pump and the curved tubing also permits a smooth exit from most arterial reservoir outlets. Attempting to fight the curve of the tubing causes twisted lines which have and can kink during cardiopulmonary bypass. Kinking during bypass can cause rupture of the line if the kink is on the positive pressure side of the pump. If the kink is on the negative side of the pump it can cause a sudden high negative pressure on the perfusate inside the tubing. Sudden negative pressure exerted on perfusate will pull gas out of solution which can coalesce into larger bubbles and, if pumped into the patient, this gas will have the same effect as emptying the arterial reservoir. Until one observes this phenomenon or experiences this accident, one is unable to fully appreciate just how much gas is contained in the perfusate in a short length of tubing.

At the present time PVC tubing presents the best tubing available to the perfusionist. The only popular alternative is silicone rubber tubing. Silicone rubber tubing evolved as a solution to the observation that red blood cells were being hemolyzed by the compression of the rollers of the roller pump or the fingers of the Sigmamotor pump. Indeed these observations were valid. However, the technology in design of the roller pump and the precision of the settings of the rollers, as well as the disappearance of the Sigmamotor pump have, by and large, eliminated this problem.

These authors do not believe that silicone rubber tubing presents a real choice to the perfusionist. The comparative biocompatability for routine cardiopulmonary bypass, less than 3 hours, has certainly not been demonstrated as being significant; however the dangers in using silicone rubber tubing are very significant.

The molecular structure of silicone rubber, along with the manufacturing process, practically guarantee that weak points will be produced and will remain in the silicone rubber tubing, and the tear resistance is low. There are no satisfactory non-destructive tests available to insure that the perfusionist will not be faced with the potential hazard of cracked or ruptured tubing. Therefore, these authors believe that silicone rubber tubing should not be used in any line in which perfusate is pumped toward the patient.

There may be some validity to the belief that silicone rubber tubing in the pumphead of the suction and vent lines reduces hemolysis. Silicone rubber tubing should not be used in the vent line if cardioplegia is pumped to the patient through the same line.

LOCKING TIES

Through the years much controversy has existed over the seemingly minor point of securing or not securing connections of the bypass circuit. Connector/tubing connections were wired together in the early years of bypass. Later connector lock nuts were developed to fit over tubing and to lock the tubing onto the connector. This device did not gain much acceptance because of the ridiculously high cost even though the idea was novel as well as practical, and the device easy to apply and remove. Self-locking nylon ties became available to perfusionists in the late 1960s. These actually came from the automobile industry and today a larger version is used as temporary handcuffs by police departments in mass arrest situations.

Concurrently the design of connectors, both integral to devices and as separate units, has improved greatly. By design, the parting line left by the two halves of the mold has been eliminated. This parting line was a ridge that extended the length of the connector, and which, on occasion was the source of air leaking into the line due to the small gap it left between the tubing and the connector. The PVC tubing could not mate tightly with the connector due to the ridge, and air was sucked under the tubing and along the ridge and into the fluid path on the tubing. With the design and manufacture of today's devices as long as the tubing is pushed on past the second barb of the connector it is secure and sealed. When pushing tubing onto a connector, the perfusionist should not grasp the tubing at the end. Holding the tubing with about three inches of the end of the tubing free is the correct way of assembling tubing to a connector. With three inches of tubing free the tubing has the ability to expand in diameter slightly as it meets resistance moving over the connector. This slight increase in diameter will facilitate moving the tubing over the connector. Connectors should never be greased or wetted in any way before applying tubing. The security of tubing on a connector depends partly on the friction at the tubing/connector interface.

Removing tubing from a connector presents a different problem. As tubing is pulled from a connector the tubing stretched and shrinks in diameter slightly, thus it grasps the connector tighter. The tubing must be prised from the tubing. This is most easily accomplished by grasping the tubing with a tubing clamp right at the end of the connector and then using the connector inside the tubing to lever against the tubing clamp. The tubing will slip down the connector a little way at first. Replace the clamp right next to the end of the connector and repeat. Tubing can usually be removed with three or four of these maneuvers.

Should tie straps be used on tubing connections today? These authors believe that as long as the tubing is applied to the dry connector correctly, that is, pushed over the second barb, tie straps are unnecessary. If a perfusionist believes he must use tie straps, then they should only be used on connections in negative pressure areas, specifically the arterial outlet of an oxygenator, for example. We believe that it is better for a connector to blow apart from over pressure, due to a clamped line or a clamp being applied while still on bypass, than for the tubing to rupture in the pumphead. The time off bypass to reconnect a connector and tubing is much shorter than to have to replace a section or whole piece of tubing and, therefore, is less hazardous to the patient. Additionally, air can be sucked into a ruptured line and pumped into the patient before the pump can be stopped. Also, if an oxygenator must be changed in the middle of cardiopulmonary bypass, undoing tie straps only adds to the time and complexity of the situation and increases the hazard to the patient.

CIRCUITS

General Conditions

The cardiopulmonary bypass circuit must be designed first with the safety of the patient in mind. The second consideration should be the adaptability of the circuit for various clinical applications and situations. The third consideration should be the ease and speed of use to the perfusionist in order to save time on a day-to-day basis and to allow for emergency set-ups. Included in the third consideration is the availability of a second perfusionist or other trained help. Circuits can be designed that permit setup by a single person while other configurations require two people. The last consideration is cost.

All tubing in the perfusion circuit should be as short as is practical and safe in order to reduce priming volume and the possible need for blood transfusion. For the same reason the diameter of the tubing should be as small as practical to accomplish adequate perfusion. However, one must take into consideration such factors as hemolysis, shear, turbulence, Reynolds number, and cavitation.

Thin wall tubing has no place in cardiopulmonary bypass. Thin wall tubing does not save money as some might imagine, thus it is not cost effective. Thin wall tubing is hazardous to the patient. It will kink more easily and can be compressed to total occlusion by the abdomen of the surgeon or assistants at the field pressing upon it. Thin wall tubing in the roller pumphead will rupture more readily and frankly, from a perfusionist's view, it is more difficult to work with. These authors recommend the use of 3/32″ thick wall tubing. Its advantages include a long track record of use without failure, acceptable levels of hemolysis, and the recommendation for its use by pump manufacturers.

Another possible safety technique that has gained popularity in recent years is the use of color-coded tubing. The tubing can be marked with stripes by the tubing manufacturer, or color tape can be applied at the time of manufacture into a custom tubing pack. The color coding on suction lines aids in communication with the surgeon. The perfusionist should be cautioned that manufacturers can make mistakes in marking tubing and perfusionists can make mistakes in assembling the perfusion circuit. Color-coding is not a very strong safety feature, but is preferable to not color-coding lines.

Some minimal debate has centered on the optimum internal diameter of tubing to be used in the arterial pumphead. Currently all adult oxygenators are manufactured with 3/8″ outlet connecters, or inlets in the case of membrane oxygenators, and most perfusionists have traditionally used 3/8″ or 5/16″ tubing through the arterial pumphead. Some few believe that large ID tubing (1/2″ or 5/8″) offer an advantage because the roller pump can be operated at a lower speed. The authors are aware of no studies that prove the beneficial effects of such practice, and the relative contributions of a properly occluded roller pump to total hemolysis during bypass is so insignificant that no rationale for this practice appears to exist.

As a general rule the fewer connections in a circuit the better. This is particularly true of the arterial line. Even though the line is under high pressure, leaks in the line can cause air to be continuously sucked into the perfusate due to the Venturi effect. This air is then pumped into the patient's arterial circulation.

Single Perfusionist Set-Up

Regardless of the design of the circuit, all tubing can be provided in a pack in a sterile condition and capped with end caps. The distal arterial and venous lines are joined together with a prebypass filter. The perfusionist assembles the circuit maintaining sterility when removing the caps from the tubing and when removing the caps from the oxygenator, or other disposable devices in the circuit and when attaching the tubing to the integral connectors of the various devices. The distal ends of the suction and vent lines are left capped. The perfusionist can prime, recirculate, filter, and debubble the oxygenator and arterial and venous lines and can check the vent and suction lines by clamping the tubing on the inlet side of the pumphead all without scrubbing, gowning, and gloving.

A second tubing pack is given to the scrub nurse which contains short lengths of tubing which are extensions of the arterial and venous lines as well as the two suction lines. These lines have connectors on the proximal ends and are capped. The scrub nurse secures these lines to the field in the appropriate place and lets the proximal ends of the tubing off the field. The perfusionist then clamps and separates the arterial and venous line, discarding the filter carefully (see Chapter 8: FILTRATION), and joins the arterial and venous line to their respective extensions onto the operating field while maintaining sterility in the process. The suction and vent lines are also connected to the extension pieces from the field in a sterile manner.

The perfusionist then can fill and recirculate through the entire arterial and venous line provided that they are joined with a connector. Direction, flow, and occlusiveness of the suction and vent lines can be determined by having the scrub nurse immerse the ends in fluid and operating the appropriate pumps. The roller heads should be operated at the speed they will be operated at during bypass. It is possible for a non-occlusive pump to suction adequately at high speed, but fail to suck at lower operational speeds. The distal ends of the arterial and venous line can be clamped and divided and the occlusion of the arterial pump set by having the scrub nurse hold up the arterial line at the level of the right atrium while the perfusionist sets the occlusion.

Using a "table pack" set-up increases the chance of loss of arterial line integrity. This places one more connector in the arterial line — one more connection that can conceivably come apart during bypass.

Two Perfusionist Set-Up

In the two person set-up one person remains sterile, scrubbed, gowned and gloved and hands off the distal capped ends of the appropriate lines to the second perfusionist who attaches the tubing to the various integral connectors in a sterile manner. The sterile perfusionist connects the arterial and venous line together with a prebypass filter. The pump is primed, recirculated, filtered, and debubbled. The suction and vent lines are checked by having the sterile person immerse the tips in fluid while the other perfusionist operates the two pumps. The sterile perfusionist clamps and separates the arterial and venous lines and unclamps and holds up the arterial line so that the perfusionist can set the arterial occlusion (a falling level of about 1 cm/min at the level of the right atrium of the patient). Then the first person takes the distal lines to the table and affixes them to the operating field in the appropriate location.

DESIGN OF CIRCUITS

Modification and variations of the different circuits discussed below exist in the practice of perfusion today. The authors will not attempt to discuss all possible circuits but rather will consider generic circuits with their various subassemblies.

Venous Line

The venous line should be thick wall, as short as possible (six feet is usually long enough), and contain no connectors, constrictions or reductions in internal diameter. The internal diameter should be appropriate to the patient size and calculated flow rate (see Table 7.1). The line should not be long enough to wrap lazily around the operating field (this is a temptation to the inexperienced at the table to clamp in a moment of boredom) or to lie on the operating room floor (where it attracts surgeons' feet like a magnet). It should be long enough to allow full-up position of the operating table without kinking at the venous inlet to the oxygenator or at any other location. It should also be long enough to allow full down positioning of the oxygenator.

Arterial Line

The arterial line should be thick-walled, as short as practical, contain as few connections as possible, and the connections in the negative pressure area of the arterial line should be externally secured with tie straps. It should be as small an internal diameter as practical for the particular patient (see Table 7.1). The arterial line should go directly to the operating field and, on the way, should drape above the venous line. It should be long enough to allow full movement of the oxygenator or table up or down without compromising the venous or arterial line connection to the oxygenator. The arterial line should not circumnavigate the operating field, but rather, should go directly from the pump to the arterial cannula.

Various ancillary equipment and monitoring devices may be operated from the arterial line with only one extra connector if proper thought and planning is given to circuit design (see Figure 7.1). As stated earlier, connections in the arterial line should be kept to the absolute minimum. Three-way stopcocks should not be used on arterial line filters or on the arterial line proper. (See Chapter 8: FILTRATION)

The arterial line is correctly the source of blood for the operation of ancillary components of the bypass circuit. A Y connector should be placed in the arterial line and all

Table 7.1 **TUBING FLUID VOLUMES**

ID Size (inches)	ml/foot (inches)
1/2	39
3/8	22
1/4	10
3/16	5

SELECTION OF LINES

Pt. Wt. (kg)	Venous ID (inches)	Arterial ID (inches)
<25	1/4*	1/4
25-65	3/8	3/8
>65	1/2	3/8

*Some protocols specify a venous line no smaller than 3/8"

other equipment, i.e., hemoconcentrator, dialyzer, sampling manifold, pressure monitor, etc. should be operated from this line. A straight connector with a luer side port should not be used as the blood source connector. The purge port of the arterial line filter should only be used to purge the filter and should remain open during bypass.

Originally suction lines were of composite diameters, usually 1/4″ ID distally and proximally with a 3/8″ ID section through the pumphead. Pediatric circuits had 1/4″ ID tubing the entire length. The reason for this configuration was that a slower RPM could be used on the roller pump with the larger diameter tubing and a larger volume of blood could be moved per unit time, giving the perfusionist an extremely large suction volume capability. With a slower RPM of the roller heads it was believed that less blood damage would occur since fewer blood formed elements would be "mashed" in the tubing between the roller and the backing plate.

The other school of thought is that the entire line should be of 1/4″ ID. Since approximately 90-95% of the open heart cases are aortocoronary bypass graft procedures which have minimal blood spillage and recovery, approximately 300 ml/case, high volume suction capability is not required. This thinking, though valid, does not provide for other types of bypass procedures which may involve large volumes of suction return such as mitral valve disease and replacement. It also does not provide for the emergency situation such as sawing into the right ventricle on a reoperation procedure where large volume suction capability will be required during cannulation.

The tubing pack design should be universal for all types of cases expected in the specific open-heart program. It should also provide for any and all emergency situations. Considerable thought should be given to the design, lest the perfusionist design himself into a corner that is not apparent until an emergency arises.

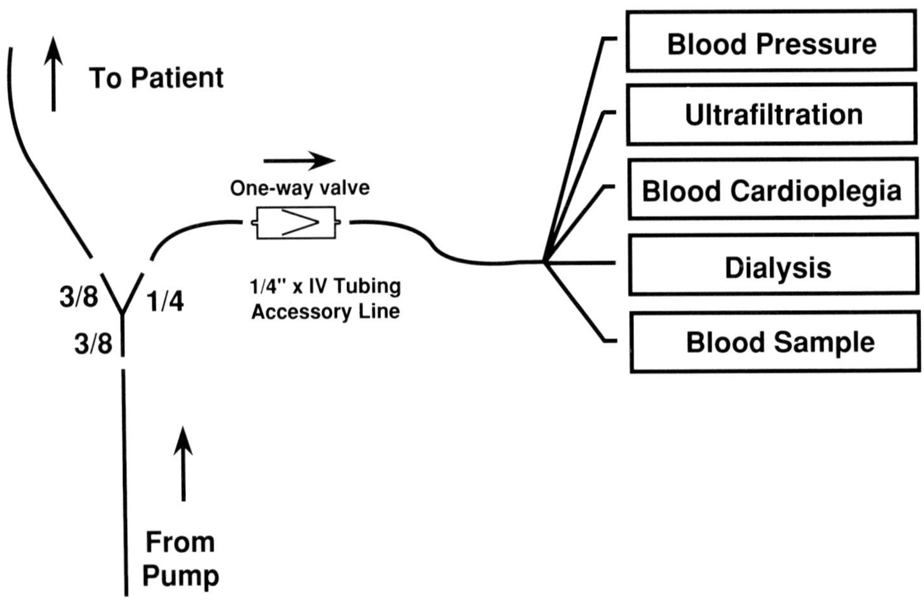

Figure 7.1. Drawing of a generic arterial line and all the possible devices which may be monitored from the line. It also shows the proper method of connecting these devices to the arterial line.

BASIC CIRCUIT DESIGN

One school of thought in designing a perfusion circuit is the one where simplicity is paramount. It holds that the simpler the circuit, the better the circuit and then fewer things that can go wrong with the circuit. Additionally, less confusion or temporary confusion is likely to occur with the simpler circuit in that the perfusionist has less to watch, and less to scan during bypass. This philosophy has a good deal of sound reasoning behind it as well as vast clinical experience.

In the most simplified cardiopulmonary bypass circuit, in addition to the oxygenator, there is an arterial and venous line, one suction line, one vent line which is also adapted and used for cardioplegia administration, and one cardiotomy reservoir with external cardiotomy filter. The reason for not simplifying further by using a filtered cardiotomy reservoir is discussed in Chapter 8: FILTRATION.

The obvious drawback to the system is the absence of an arterial line filter. Recent evidence indicates utilization of this device is prudent perfusion practice, particularly if used properly with a passively purging line affixed to the filter purge port. Consequently, the simplest circuit should contain an arterial line filter without filter bypass line and with purge line returning to the oxygenator (see Figure 7.2). In a life-threatening emergency the arterial filter should be eliminated from the arterial line to save the priming and debubbling time.

Another minor limitation of the simple circuit is the use of a single vent line to both decompress the heart and administer cardioplegic solution. In situations where only one injection of cardioplegia is the practice, this set-up is not limiting, but in situations where multiple injections of cardioplegia are given during the procedure, the venting function must be stopped for a period of time while cardioplegia is administered, which might be long enough to cause over-distention of the myocardium with subsequent damage to that tissue.

From this basic circuit the perfusionist may add any number of ancillary devices such as hemoconcentrator, a dialyzer, or a cardioplegia delivery system, etc. Safety devices and circuits may also be added to the design. Those designed to prevent massive air emboli are recommended for the arterial portion of the circuit. All types of monitoring devices are readily incorporated into the design. Figure 7.3 shows most of the possibilities available to the perfusionist in composite form.

Regardless of the complexity of the cardiopulmonary bypass circuit, the perfusionist should arrange all components of the circuit for maximum visibility and efficiency of movement. For example, the oxygenator reservoir should always be optimally visible and protected from any traffic around the pump. The arterial pumphead should be as close to the oxygenator as possible. The gas flow meters are manipulated less frequently than the pump speed control knob, so they can be located away from the oxygenator. If the system includes an anesthetic vaporizer then it is even more important to locate it away from the oxygenator. Disastrous results of leaking volatile fluids on polycarbonate components have been reported.

Because correct vent operation is crucial in deairing the heart, the vent pumphead should be located next to the arterial pump. Problems associated with the continual satisfactory function of the vent can be alleviated by inserting a 25 ga. needle proximal to the vent entering the heart or the use of an in-line vent valve which will prevent positive pressure to the patient as well as automatically releasing excessive negative pressure.

If the perfusionist administers cardioplegia by pump it also should be located near at hand. Pressure monitors and cardioplegia reservoirs for cardioplegia should be located together to facilitate visual monitoring. The arterial pressure monitor should not be located adjacent to the cardioplegia pressure monitor to avoid confusion between the two devices.

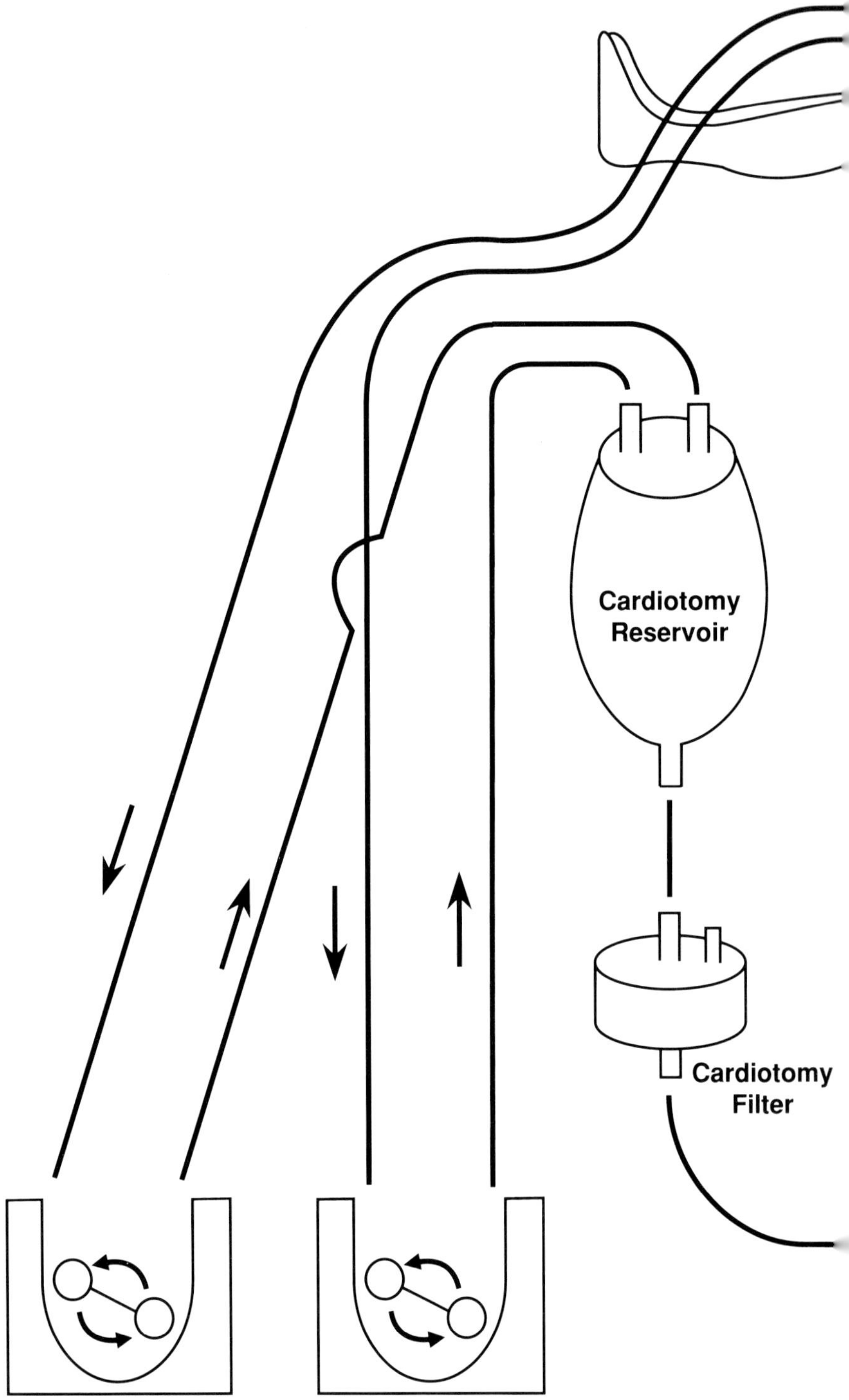
Cardiotomy
Reservoir
Cardiotomy
Filter

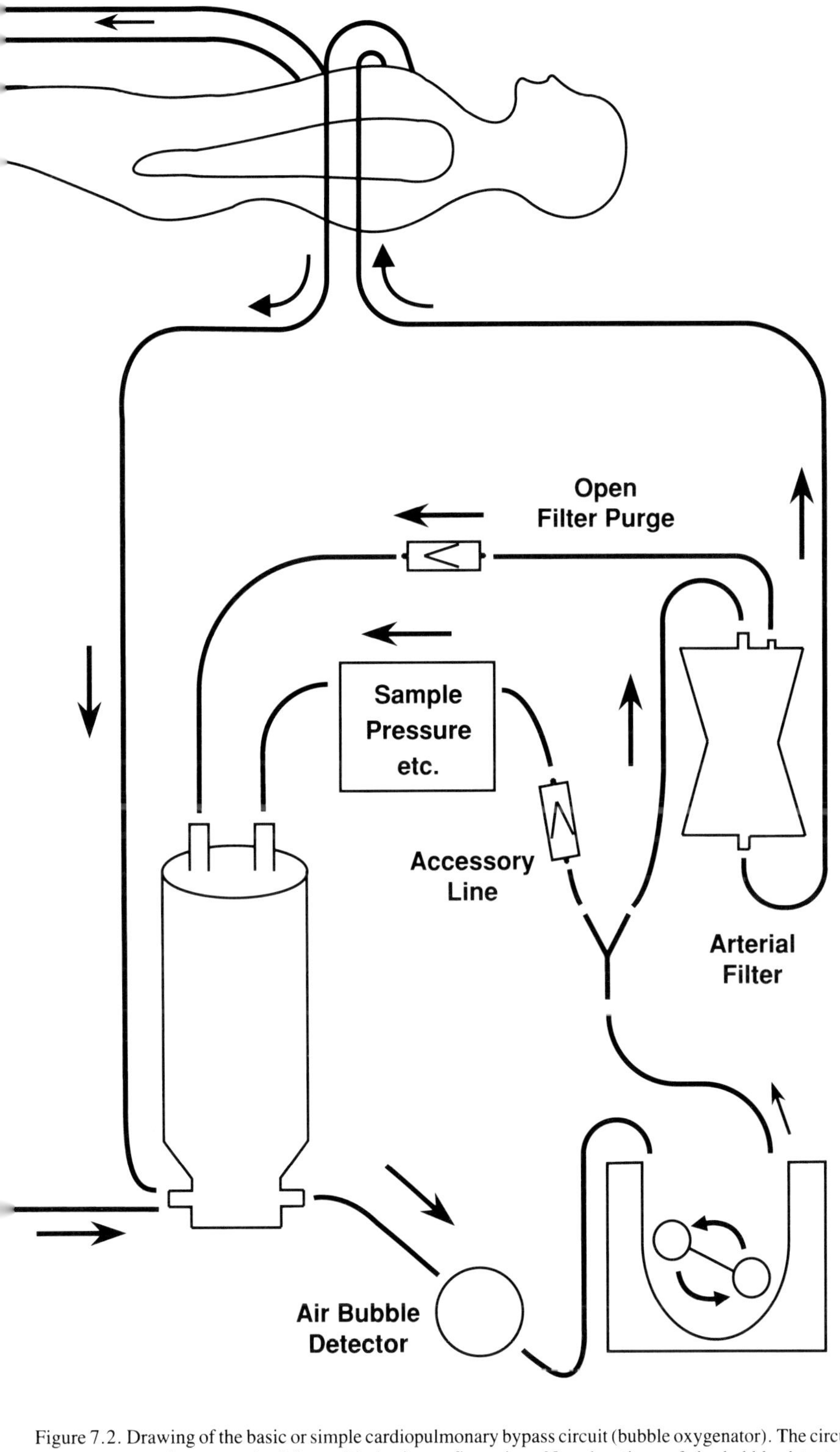

Figure 7.2. Drawing of the basic or simple cardiopulmonary bypass circuit (bubble oxygenator). The circuit design may be customized from this basic configuration. Note locations of the bubble detector and the one-way valve in the arterial filter purge line.

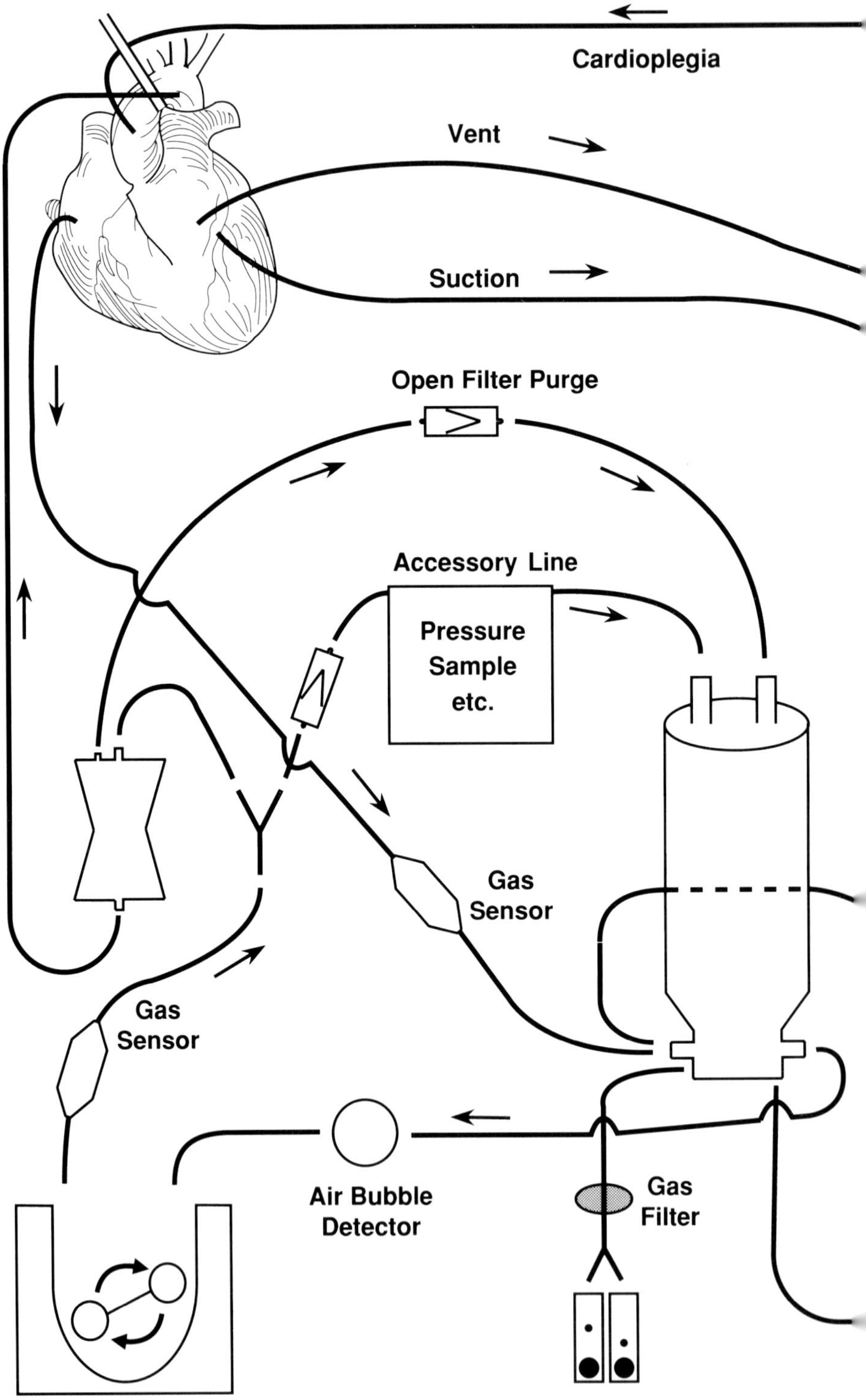
Cardioplegia
Vent
Suction
Open Filter Purge
Accessory Line
Pressure
Sample
etc.
Gas
Sensor
Gas
Sensor
Air Bubble
Detector
Gas
Filter

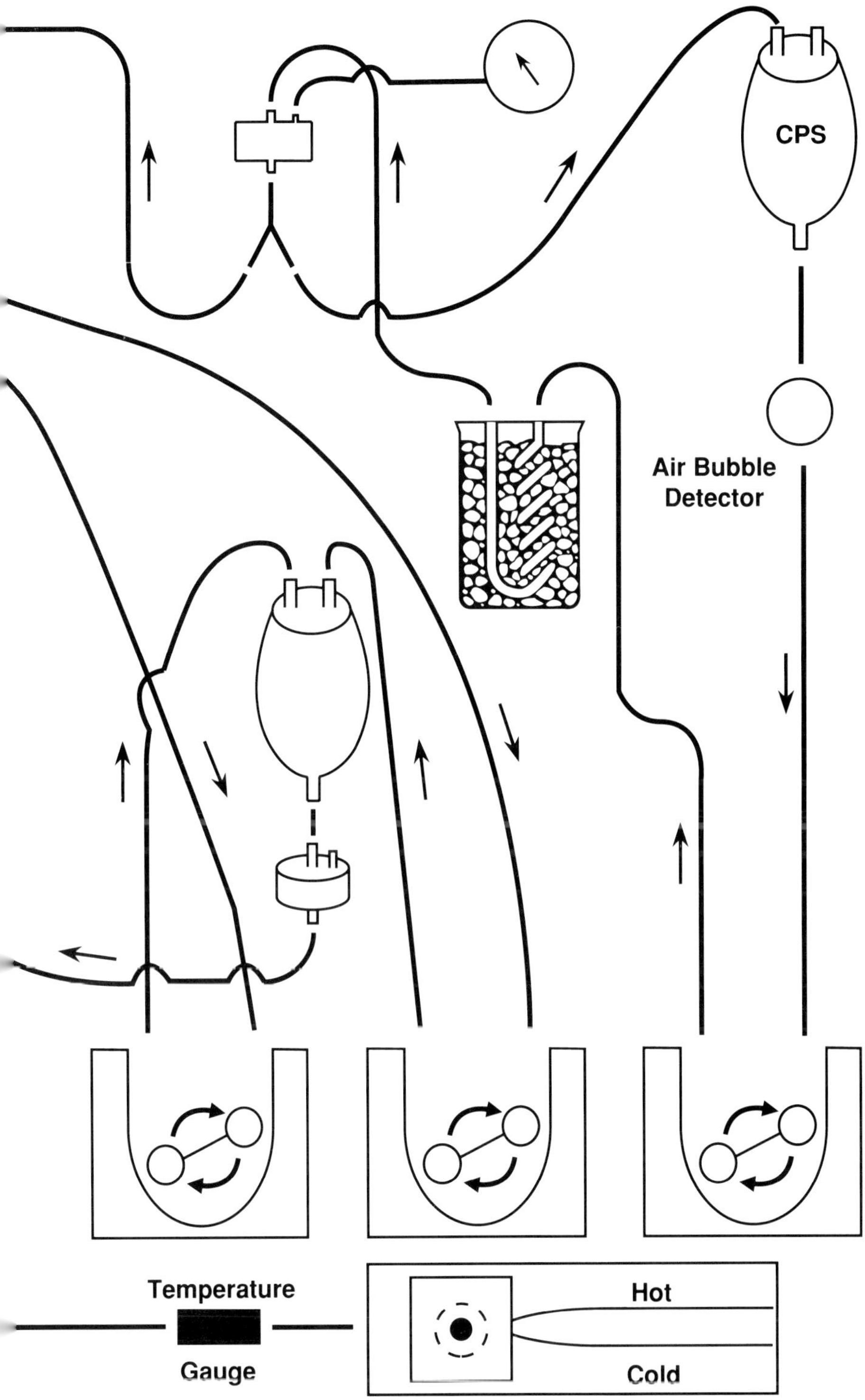

Figure 7.3. Drawing of a composite cardiopulmonary bypass circuit which incorporates most of the possible equipment that could be added to the circuit. The proper locations and methods of connection are also shown.

The least important pumphead is the pump sucker. It can be located the farthest from the perfusionist.

Once an ultrafiltration device is filled with blood, its operation consists of simply clamping or unclamping the ultrafiltrate drain line depending upon whether one wants it to function or not. Blood can be passively shunted through the device from the accessory line from the arterial line Y. Thus the ultrafiltration device can be located somewhat away from the perfusionist with the compromise of increased volume requirements with increased distance.

All other patient perfusion parameter monitors should be located conveniently to the visual scanning pattern of the perfusionist. The perfusionist's attention should never be drawn too far from the arterial reservoir level.

Every separate component of the cardiopulmonary bypass circuit should be readily available in the operating room as a separate and sterile item for use in an emergency. This includes separate arterial and venous lines as well as suction lines. A wide variety of connectors, reducers, and Y connectors and short lengths of 1/4″, 3/8″ and 1/2″ ID tubing should be available as separate and sterile items whether they are routinely used or not.

..LAWSUITS AND ... CASENOTES

.. A 34 year-old engineer with a family of four underwent cardiopulmonary bypass for aortocoronary bypass graft surgery. Forty minutes into the procedure air bubbles were observed in the coronary grafts by the surgeon. Upon examination of the bypass circuit, a small crack was found in the silicone rubber arterial line and was located in the pumphead section of the circuit. During the negative pressure phase of the roller head air was sucked into the arterial line and pumped into the patient. There was no way of determining when during bypass the crack occurred, and consequently there was no way of determining how much air had been infused or for how long. The patient was essentially brain dead. Liability was disavowed by the hospital for the contract perfusionist. The case was settled out of court for an undisclosed amount. The hospital did pay for the perfusionist's share of the settlement.

.. During cardiopulmonary bypass the oxygenator fell or was knocked from the oxygenator holder bracket. When the oxygenator struck the operating room floor the arterial line fell off of the arterial outlet connector. Air was sucked into the arterial line and pumped into the arterial circulation of the patient who was pronounced dead on the operating table after the successful completion of the scheduled operative procedure. A malpractice suit was filed against the perfusionist, hospital, surgeon, and oxygenator manufacturer. The suit was settled out of court for an undisclosed amount.

... Thin-walled PVC tubing was being used in the arterial pumphead with a new pump. The team was accustomed to using this type tubing and had performed several thousand cases. In the middle of bypass the arterial pumphead tubing ruptured. Air from the arterial line was successfully vented out the arterial filter purge line. The ruptured tubing was replaced and bypass continued. There was no patient injury. The exact complication occurred in another case a few days later with the same results. Inspection of the heart-lung machine revealed a sharp edge on the outflow side of the backing plate. The thin-walled tubing rode up in the raceway during bypass and was split by the roller action pressing it against the sharp edge. The perfusionist is now using 3/32″ wall tubing which does not ride up in the raceway. The manufacturer subsequently redesigned the pump.

... Silicone rubber tubing in the arterial pumphead abruptly split during cardiopulmonary bypass. No bubble trap or arterial filter was being used, and the patient received a massive air embolism and subsequently died. Examination of the silicone tubing revealed no apparent flaws. Further investigation revealed that the tubing manufacturer had changed the formulation which greatly increased the susceptibility of the silicone rubber tubing to tearing during repeated flexing.

Chapter 8:

FILTRATION

Chapter 8: FILTRATION

GAS

Gas line filters are used to prevent bacterial contamination and debris from metal tanks of compressed gas being blown into the cardiopulmonary bypass circuit. A gas line filter is placed in the low pressure gas line between the flow meter or blender and the oxygenator gas inlet. The filter is placed some distance away from the oxygenator in the gas line to avoid contact with priming fluid or blood if gas flow is interrupted. If accidentally wetted, the gas line filter can restrict gas flow causing decreased oxygenation or gas line rupture during bypass. Some gas line filters are marked with the direction of gas flow and must be incorporated in the bypass circuit in the proper direction. Reversing the direction of gas flow through a gas line filter also can restrict gas flow. Gas line filters are designed for one time use only.

PREBYPASS

Prebypass filters are available in several rated pore sizes from 5 microns to 0.2 microns. The purpose of prebypass filtration is to remove particulate debris from the cardiopulmonary bypass circuit. The source of such particulate debris is primarily from the manufacturing process of disposable devices, although some particulates may be air- borne in origin, generated during assembly of the circuit, or contained in priming fluids.

Prebypass filtration usually is accomplished by inserting a prebypass filter at the arterial-venous connection between the two lines. During crystalloid priming and recirculation, particulate debris is washed out of the entire bypass circuit and trapped in the prebypass filter. The prebypass filter is removed and discarded before adding any blood products to the circuit.

To properly wash a hard-shell type oxygenator thoroughly, more crystalloid than would normally be necessary to prime the circuit is added. This raises the fluid level in the reservoir which wets and rinses those parts of the oxygenator that later may be exposed to blood during cardiopulmonary bypass with higher blood reservoir levels. 2000 to 3000 ml is sufficient for most simple adult circuits.

The optimum duration and rate of flow for prebypass filtration has not been established, but an early study would suggest more effective removal of particulates with longer (i.e., >30 minutes) recirculation times.[1] However, longer recirculation times may not be practical, and these can be circumvented by higher recirculation flow rates for shorter periods of time. Prebypass filtration is performed early during the set-up while other parts of the cardiopulmonary bypass system are assembled. Prebypass recirculation is performed continuously for five to ten minutes at 5/L minute flow on all adult cases. For pediatric set-ups, the flow rate is 2.5 L/min for five to ten minutes.

When the prebypass filter is removed, care should be taken not to allow trapped particulates to inadvertently reenter the circuit by inverting the filter during its removal. This also can be prevented by clamping the tubing just proximally and distally before removing the prebypass filter. Any crystalloid remaining in the filter and discarded should be accounted for when recording the volume of perfusate or in calculating patient hemodilutional effects. In most prebypass filters, this volume is miniscule, but with large surface area and finer pore-sized filters this may account for up to 50 cc.

CARDIOTOMY

Filtration of "cardiotomy" or suctioned blood is accomplished by an external filter located in the cardiotomy drainage line or an integral filter in the cardiotomy reservoir.

Some oxygenators incorporate an integral cardiotomy filter thus eliminating the need for a separate reservoir. Several studies have reported the beneficial effects of filtration of cardiotomy blood which contains platelet aggregates, cell fragments, fat, and tissue debris from the operative site.[2-4] Cardiotomy filters must be able to handle blood, air, and foam at variable and intermittent flow rates. Hold-up of cardiotomy suctioned blood should be minimal, particularly during pediatric perfusion. One technique to decrease hold-up volume is to pre-wet the cardiotomy filter with crystalloid solution. This is easily accomplished at the time of circuit priming by administration of crystalloid through the cardiotomy reservoir. The cardiotomy filter should not be allowed to dry out before or during cardiopulmonary bypass to decrease the likelihood of cardiotomy filter blockage.

Occasionally, a cardiotomy filter may become blocked, especially if the pump suckers are used before adequate heparin anticoagulation or following bypass after protamine has been administered. Another possible cause of a blocked cardiotomy filter is if blood is allowed to pool for prolonged periods in the cardiotomy filter. Suctioning of cryoprecipitate ("fibrin glue") from the operative field with subsequent clotting in the cardiotomy reservoir also has occurred. Since a blocked integral filter in a cardiotomy reservoir can be hazardous to the patient, it would seem preferable to use a non-filtered reservoir with an external extracorporeal filter that can be changed out with ease, a practice these authors endorse. However, the majority of perfusionists appear to use a filtered cardiotomy reservoir according to survey data.[5]

When a filtered cardiotomy reservoir becomes blocked, the perfusionist's instinct simply may be to pressurize the reservoir occluding the vent and using the sucker as an air pressure source, overcome the blockage, and continue on with cardiopulmonary bypass. *These authors are unalterably opposed to this technique of pressurizing the cardiotomy at any time for any reason.* If this blockage occurs, the reservoir should be changed out and the blood recovered from the first reservoir and admitted into the new reservoir for filtration and debubbling.

Using the technique of pressurization of the reservoir at best will extrude aggregates and debris the diameter of the filter mesh in the filtered cardiotomy reservoir filter. This debris may well aggregate downstream into larger aggregates and clots which may compromise the oxygenator itself. At worst, using this technique may cause a gas embolism to be introduced into the patient's aorta,[6] or alternatively, rupture of the perfusion circuit with resultant blood loss and the necessity for stopping bypass abruptly while a new circuit is assembled and replaced.

Following cardiopulmonary bypass if the cardiotomy reservoir with integral filter is converted to a chest tube drainage autotransfusion reservoir,[7] appropriate sterile tubing connections are added to functionally make this conversion (see Chapter 21: AUTOTRANSFUSION).

While chest tube drainage blood usually contains few viable platelets or clotting factors, the time required for its reinfusion may be prolonged and highly variable in the ICU due to different rates of bleeding. Under these circumstances, some clotting still can occur in the converted cardiotomy reservoir. To prevent infusion of these clots, a blood filter may be added below the reservoir in line with the infusion pump.

ARTERIAL

Arterial line filters are used to remove both particulate and gaseous microemboli before arterial blood is returned to the patient's systemic circulation. A very important secondary benefit is that an arterial filter will usually function as a gross bubble trap if large volumes of gas accidentally enter the arterial line.

Currently, arterial line filtration is used by four out of five perfusionists, and the vast majority of arterial line filters used are of the screen type.[5] Safe use of an arterial line filter is dependent on proper priming, operation with an open one-way purge line, and maintenance of adequate blood anticoagulation during bypass which is generally assessed by the activated clotting time (ACT).

Priming an arterial filter is facilitated by carbon dioxide purging prior to filling the filter with crystalloid. The purge gas is filtered by a gas line filter and is administered either directly into the filter via the vent port or via a sampling line port connected to the filter. If a closed membrane oxygenator system is used, any port in the arterial-venous circuit may be used for introduction of purge gas. It is important that the CO_2 gas thoroughly permeates the filter medium to displace air. A recent study has shown that six minutes of CO_2 purging at 6 L/minute is adequate to remove virtually all residual air from an arterial filter.[8]

Once the filter is CO_2 purged, crystalloid solution is slowly pumped into the filter. If a filter bypass line is used, the filter is primed in a retrograde fashion. If no bypass line is used, antegrade priming is used. It is important that the purge line is open during priming so that gas is vented out as crystalloid fills the filter.

It is not necessary to completely debubble the arterial filter during the prebypass wash and recirculation. However, after the prebypass filter is removed and any blood products are added to the circuit, the arterial filter is thoroughly debubbled by recirculating, tapping, rotating and inverting the filter. High flow rates with normal circuit pressures aid debubbling, as does intermittently restricting and releasing the arterial line on the outlet side. The momentary increase/decrease in pressure in the filter housing will dislodge remaining gas bubbles. Use of salt poor albumin or blood in the perfusate also aids debubbling due to surface tension effects, but these are not absolutely necessary for proper debubbling of an arterial line filter.

Adequacy of filter debubbling is assessed visually by stopping flow, inverting the filter and tapping the housing. If no bubbles are seen to rise into the outlet tubing, one is reasonably assured the filter is adequately debubbled. If bubbles are observed to exit from the filter, the process should be repeated until no visible bubbles are seen exiting the filter.

During bypass the filter is held stationary at a low point in the cardiopulmonary bypass set-up with the purge or vent port uppermost. A one-way valved purge line is connected to the filter in such a way that *no stopcocks are attached to the filter*. This technique lessens the risk of either accidentally admitting air into the filter or leaking blood. The one-way valve is positioned to allow flow *out* of the filter only (see Figure 8.1).

The arterial filter purge line drains back into the oxygenator at a low pressure site, preferably in the pre-defoamer section, as any restriction to purge line flow can compromise its effectiveness. If a closed membrane oxygenator system is used the purge line is drained into the venous line.

Prior to establishing bypass, the purge line stopcock is closed to maintain arterial line integrity. Upon establishing pump flow, the purge line stopcock is opened to allow a small volume of the arterial blood to continuously shunt out of the filter. This provides a low pressure vent for gaseous microemboli or gross air embolism. Use of an open arterial filter purge line is not a fool proof safety technique, however, as gross air can be pumped through a vented arterial filter if the volumes and pressures exceed the venting capabilities and bubble point pressure of the filter.[9] Use of a continuously purging arterial line filter should be used with caution during pediatric perfusion and is contraindicated during infant perfusion where the shunted blood flow is proportionally much higher in relation to arterial pump flow. Purge line flow generally is 200 to 400 ml/minute but may be as high as 500-700 ml/minute depending on arterial line pressure, the size of the purge line and stopcocks, and presence or absence of a one-way valve.

The necessity of having to use an arterial filter bypass line with current screen arterial line filters is rarely required.[5] This practice evolved during early clinical experience when depth type arterial line filters were used and less than adequate heparinization was commonplace. Cases of thrombus forming during bypass or in the arterial filter bypass line have been reported.[10,11] Isolating the arterial filter by opening a bypass line to maintain blood flow would likely transmit emboli to the patient under these conditions. The only alternative to correct an occluded arterial line filter if no bypass line is used is to stop bypass and remove the filter. If it is determined that only the arterial filter is blocked, then it can be quickly replaced with a sterile straight connector. During any such emergent removal of the arterial filter, extreme care must be taken to exclude all air when the arterial line is reconnected. This can be accomplished by forming a meniscus of blood as the tubing is inserted over the connector.

A worse situation is if gross clotting occurs in the oxygenator. This may not always be visible or apparent to the perfusionist, but clots formed in the oxygenator can embolize to the arterial filter and eventually occlude it. The only alternative in this situation is to stop cardiopulmonary bypass and change out the entire circuit including arterial and venous lines and oxygenator. Because of the time required to adequately prime and debubble an arterial filter, it should be eliminated under these emergency conditions. A disposable bubble trap can be used in place of the arterial filter and it is easily primed and debubbled. Alternatively, bypass can continue with neither a filter or bubble trap in the arterial line.

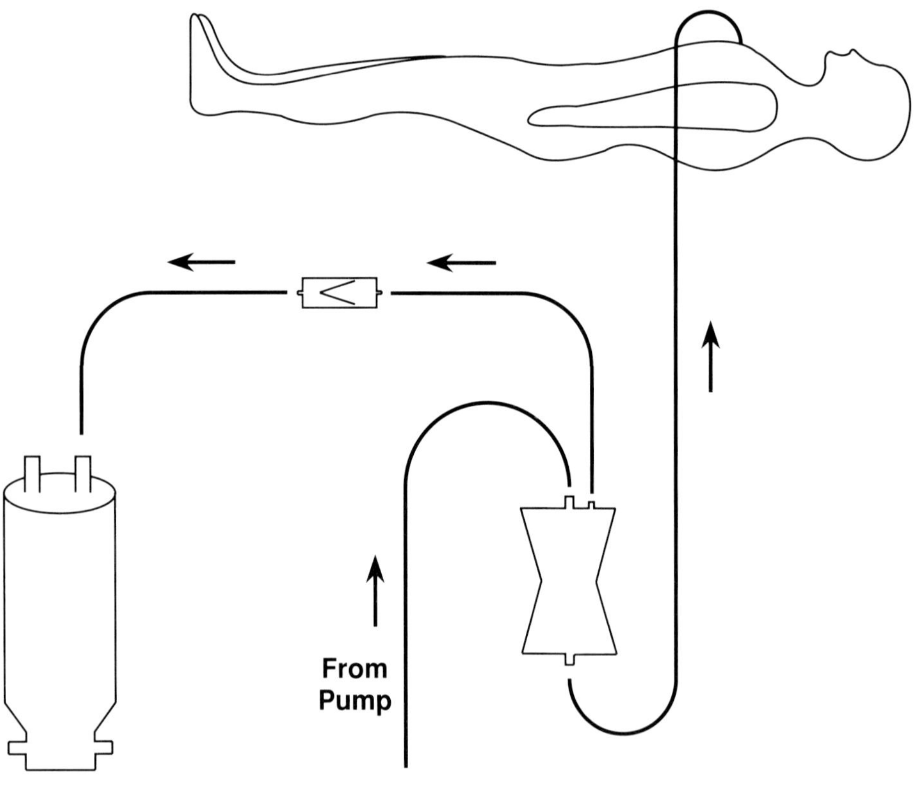

Figure 8.1 Connection of arterial filter one-way valved purge line to low pressure site in oxygenator. Note that no stopcocks are placed on the arterial filter.

A Y connector with an accessory line (Figure 8.2) should serve as the source for arterial line pressure monitoring, ultrafiltration, blood sampling site, or whatever.

With current management of cardiopulmonary bypass anticoagulation with ACTs, the arterial filter bypass line reasonably can be eliminated from the bypass set-up. While all arterial line filter manufacturers' instructions recommend incorporation of a bypass line, both the rationale for and the clinical frequency of its use support its elimination from the bypass circuit, a practice which these authors endorse.

Directly measuring the pressure drop across an arterial filter without a bypass line is not possible. However from a practical standpoint, knowing what the pressure is in the arterial line before the arterial filter and the patient's arterial, or perfusion pressure does allow one to approximate the arterial filter pressure drop. If the arterial line pressure abruptly increases with no change or a decrease in the patient's perfusion pressure, the arterial cannula or line may be malpositioned or kinked. Likewise, if the patient's systemic vascular resistance increases, the arterial line pressure will increase which *does not* signify an occluded arterial line filter. Significant and abrupt increases in the arterial line pressure are most often due to hemodynamic causes as described above. Blockage of an arterial line filter occurs only rarely and is manifested by a significant gradual rise in the arterial line pressure without a corresponding rise in the patient's perfusion pressure. Figures 8.3a & b show the techniques for measuring arterial line pressure and pressure drop across an arterial filter.

ULTRAFILTRATION

Ultrafiltration (also called hemoconcentration) is the controlled removal of plasma water and solutes from blood by molecular filtration. It is an ideal technique for cardiopulmonary bypass in heparinized patients because of easy access to blood removal and return sites. It is used to lessen the effects of hemodilution during bypass either from non-blood primes or administration of cardioplegic solution. Ultrafiltration is accomplished by shunt-

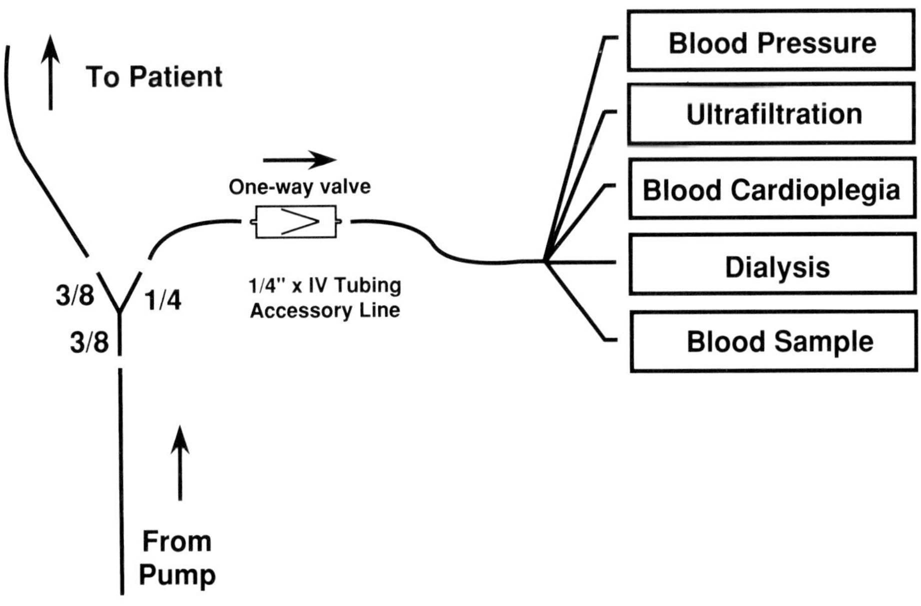

Figure 8.2 Arterial line Y with pre-attached purge or access line.

ing blood through an ultrafiltration device at relatively low flows (<500 ml/minute) and at sufficient pressures as are found in the arterial line. Ultrafiltration, or plasma water removal rates depend on the blood flow through the device, pressure drop, hydrostatic pressure in the ultrafiltrate line, and hematocrit. Elevated values of these parameters, except for hematocrit, increase the ultrafiltration rates which generally range from 15 to 75 ml/minute (average range 25-45 ml/minute). Patients with lower hematocrits also exhibit greater ultrafiltration rates.

Ultrafiltration devices are rinsed with one to two liters of sterile, normal saline prior to placement in the bypass circuit to remove glycerine which has been added at the time of manufacture.

Blood may be either pumped through the ultrafiltration device or passively shunted through from the arterial line. The arterial accessory line provides a simple source of blood for the ultrafiltration device. However, it is important that the perfusionist increase the arterial flow to compensate for blood shunted through the ultrafiltration device. Once blood flow is established through the ultrafiltration device, it is maintained to avoid stasis and possible plugging. Removal of plasma water is controlled by clamping or unclamping the ultrafiltration drain line. Criterion for initiating ultrafiltration include a large oxygenator reservoir blood volume and a low hematocrit. The ultrafiltration device also is used

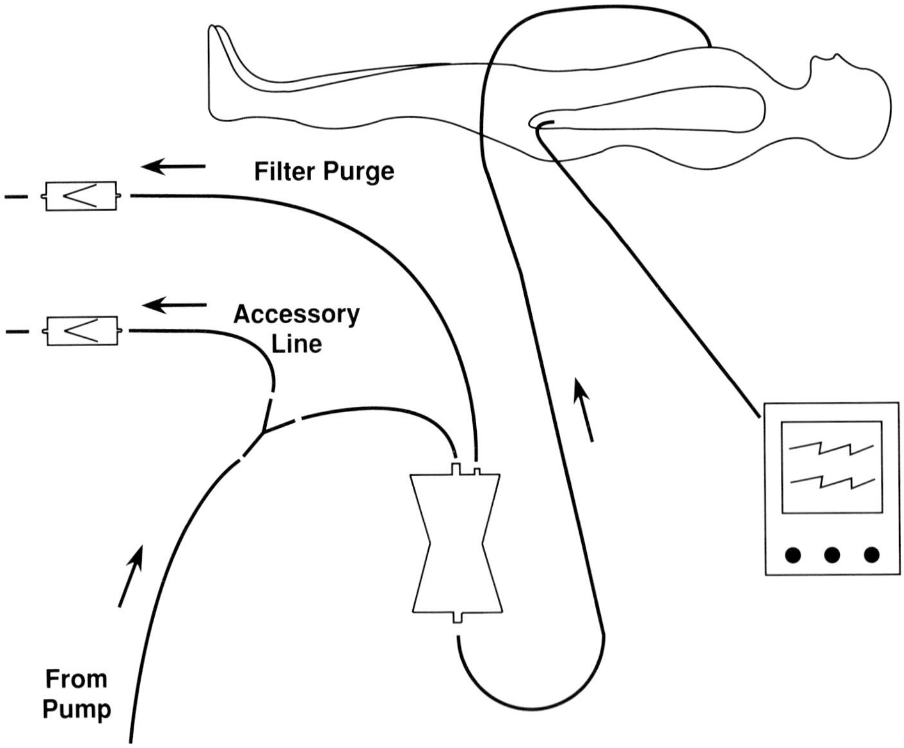

Figure 8.3a Standard arterial line configuration with no filter bypass line. Pressure monitor connected to the arterial line Y displays arterial line pressure before the filter. The patient's radial artery pressure is displayed on an electronic monitor along with ECG and other pressures. Pressure drop across the filter can only be approximated.

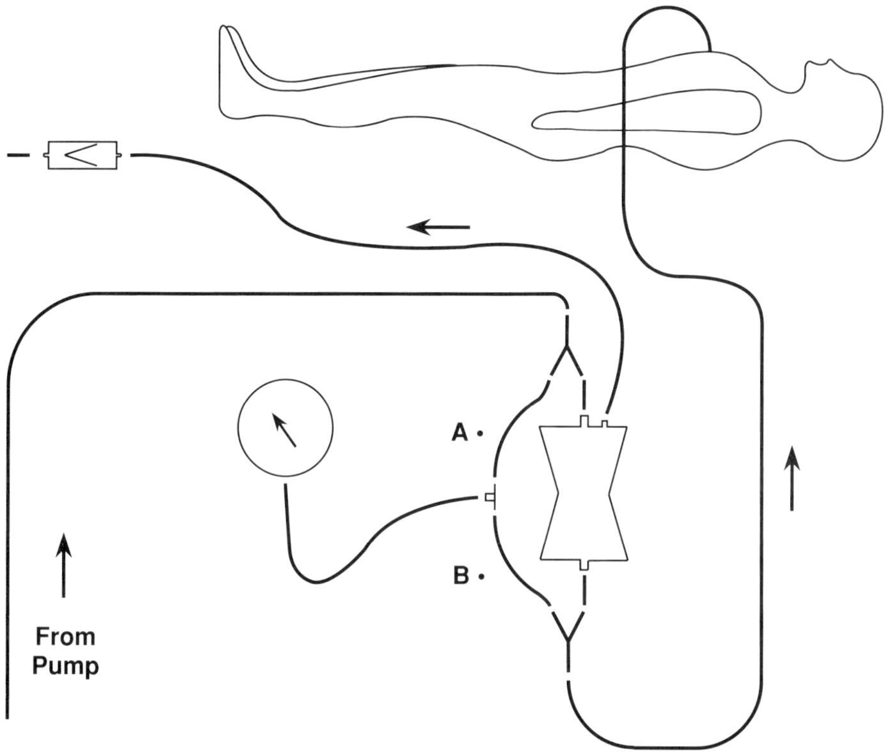

Figure 8.3b Alternative technique for measuring ΔP across an arterial filter without diverting blood flow through the bypass line. A straight connector with a luer port is incorporated in the bypass line. By moving the bypass line clamp either proximal (point A) or distal (point B) to the connector, upstream or downstream pressures will be monitored. Note that no one-way valved line is used in the pressure monitor line, and use of this technique should only be to a closed, fluid-filled pressure monitoring system to avoid air embolism when changing clamps.

following bypass to concentrate blood remaining in the circuit. A rough guide for the hematocrit of concentrated blood is that halving the volume of blood remaining in the cardiopulmonary bypass circuit will double its hematocrit.

CARDIOPLEGIA

Crystalloid cardioplegia consists of stock crystalloid solution with additives (e.g., potassium, mannitol, dextrose). Cardioplegia solution may be commercially manufactured, prepared by the hospital pharmacy, or mixed by operating room personnel just prior to use. The process of adding drugs to stock crystalloid solution generates particulates. Large surface area, sub-micron pore-sized filters are available to remove particulates from cardioplegic solution before it is administered to the patient's heart. Deleterious effects of such particulates on the coronary vasculature have been shown in one study using the rat heart model.[12]

If the cardioplegia filter is placed in the delivery line, the pressure drop across the filter must be known if one wishes to accurately control the aortic root or coronary perfusion pressure. For cardioplegia delivery systems in the cardiopulmonary bypass circuit where volume is not limited, a 0.2 micron prebypass filter is used because of low pressure drop (<50 mmHg @ 500 ml/minute flow) (see Chapter 18: MYOCARDIAL PROTECTION).

Cold crystalloid cardioplegia solution with dextrose is more viscous than room temperature crystalloid, and the pressure drop will be greater than solutions containing no dextrose.

An added advantage of a cardioplegia filter in the delivery line is prevention of gas embolism. According to The Survey data, aortic root air during administration of cardioplegic solution was the second most frequently observed type of gas embolism during cardiopulmonary bypass.

If blood cardioplegia is used, obviously, a submicron pore-sized filter cannot be used. A conventional extracorporeal blood filter (20 to 40 micron pore size) is used to remove blood aggregates and also will act as a bubble trap.

BUBBLE TRAPS

Bubble traps for the arterial line were used on early bypass set- ups due to the high risk of morbidity or mortality associated with gross systemic air embolism. These early bubble traps were non- disposable, had no provision for continuous venting of smaller bubbles, and were considered generally effective for capturing large volumes of gas that accidentally entered the arterial line.

Screen arterial blood filters also function as effective bubble traps, and recent survey respondents noted the primary benefit of arterial filtration was for the removal of either gross air emboli or gaseous microemboli.[5] Until recently there were few bubble traps commercially available. However, the authors are aware of five models in use at the present time, despite there being no studies evaluating their efficacy. Until such time as these studies are forthcoming, disposable bubble traps offer the perfusionist a less expensive alternative to an arterial line filter in decreasing the risk of gross air embolism from the arterial line (see Chapter 26: AIR).

REFERENCES

1. Brooks JD, Beauchamp RA, Magrath RA and Clark RE: Efficacy of particulate removal by a pre-bypass filter with different oxygenation systems. JECT 11:175, 1979.
2. Solis RT, Noon GP, Beall Jr AC and DeBakey ME: Particulate microembolism during cardiac operation. Ann Thorac Surg 17:332, 1974.
3. Solis RT, Kennedy PS, Beall Jr AC, Noon GP and DeBakey ME: Cardiopulmonary bypass, microembolization and platelet aggregation. Circulation 52:103, 1975.
4. Clark RE, Margraf HW and Beauchamp RA: Fat and solid filtration in clinical perfusions. Surg 77:216, 1975.
5. Kurusz M, Schneider B, Brown JP and Conti VR: Filtration during open-heart surgery: Devices, techniques, opinions and complications. Proceed Am Acad Cardiovasc Perfusion 4:123, 1983.
6. Mills NL and Ochsner JL: Massive air embolism during cardiopulmonary bypass: Causes, prevention, and management. J Thorac Cardiovasc Surg 80:708, 1980.
7. Cosgrove DM, Amiot DM and Meserko JJ: An improved technique for autotransfusion of shed mediastinal blood. Ann Thorac Surg 40:519, 1985.
8. Hargrove M, McCarthy AP and Fitzpatrick GJ: Carbon dioxide flushing prior to priming the bypass circuit; An experimental derivation of the optimal flow rate and duration of the flushing process. Perfusion 2:177, 1987.
9. Pascale F: Removal of gaseous microemboli from extracorporeal circulation. Med Instrument 19:70, 1985.
10. Hardin SB: Case reports: Thrombus formation in the extracorporeal circuit. JECT 16:27, 1984.
11. Clark DC, Thompson JD, Brannon H and Owens G: Idiopathic fibrin formation within the extracorporeal circuit. Proceed Am Acad Cardiovasc Perfusion 5:150, 1984.
12. Robinson LA, Braimbridge MV and Hearse DJ: The potential hazard of particulate contamination of cardioplegic solutions. J Thorac Cardiovasc Surg 87:48, 1984.

..LAWSUITS AND ...CASENOTES

.. During cardiopulmonary bypass for aortocoronary bypass graft surgery the perfusionist allowed the arterial reservoir to empty and air was pumped into the patient. An arterial line filter was being used in the arterial line but the stopcock was closed. No other safety devices were in use. The patient died several days later. Suit was filed against the perfusionist, the hospital, the surgeons, and the anesthesiologist. The case was settled out of court for an amount in excess of $225,000.

.. During cardiopulmonary bypass the perfusionist allowed the arterial reservoir to empty when the surgeon inadvertently temporarily occluded the venous return line. Air was pumped into the patient, who subsequently died. An arterial line filter was part of the set-up, however the perfusionist was using the purge port to measure filter pressure and no purge line returned to the oxygenator or reservoir. A low level sensing device was in use but failed to function properly. Suit was filed against the perfusionist, hospital, and surgeon. The case settled out of court for an amount in excess of $350,000.

.. The open-heart team had changed to a different arterial line filter and experienced a sudden and unexplained rise in postoperative neurological complications. They stopped using the new filter and the perfusionist told the hospital and surgeon that he would have the filters tested by an independent laboratory. He was then assured by the manufacturer that his was the first complaint concerning the filter and that in-house tests by the manufacturer revealed no irregularities with the filters he had returned. He did not seek outside testing or evaluation of the filters in question as he had assured the hospital and surgeon that he would. Of his own volition he resumed use of the arterial line filter in question. The team experienced a resumption of the unexplained neurological complications. Two occurred on consecutive patients on the same day. Neurological sequelae included brain death, on one extreme, through blindness, to transient neurological problems on the other end of the spectrum. Three separate lawsuits were filed by three separate plaintiffs. Two cases were settled out of court for an undisclosed amount. The third suit settled out of court against the perfusionist, the hospital, and the surgeon for an amount in excess of $50,000. The suit continued to trial against the manufacturer of the arterial line filter. The judge dismissed the case on motion by the manufacturer holding that the plaintiff had not proved that the filter was the proximate cause of the brain damage suffered by the plaintiff. The case was not appealed.

... The perfusionist had used an arterial line filter and had an open purge line which returned to the cardiotomy reservoir. During the bypass procedure the cardiotomy reservoir was inadvertently pressurized. Air was forced retrograde into the filter and then into the arterial line and into the patient. The patient died on the second postoperative day.

... At the start of cardiopulmonary bypass the surgeon noted a surge of air through the arterial line and into the patient. Bypass was stopped and the circuit inspected after attempts to remove all air from the patient. Inspection revealed a three way stopcock on the purge port which was open to air. The patient died the following day.

... The coronary artery bypass graft operation was complete and the perfusionist was rewarming the patient at full flow. The surgeon lifted the heart to inspect the circumflex artery anastomosis, and venous return from a single atrial cannula was briefly interrupted. The perfusionist did not notice the abrupt decrease in the level of the arterial reservoir which was depleted in less than ten seconds. A massive volume of air entered the arterial line before the perfusionist heard the unusual sound. The pump was immediately stopped but air entered the arterial filter where it was vented out the open purge line. No air was observed distal to the arterial line filter. After a few seconds off bypass to refill and debubble the arterial line, bypass was resumed and then discontinued uneventfully after the patient had been rewarmed. The patient made a normal postoperative recovery.

... NOTE
Numerous cases of air emboli retrograde through the purge line from a pressurized cardiotomy reservoir and air emboli in which the purge vent port was not open have been reported with results from no sequelae to brain death.

Chapter 9:

BLOOD PUMPS AND PULSATILE PERFUSION

Chapter 9: BLOOD PUMPS AND PULSATILE PERFUSION

In the history of cardiopulmonary bypass many types of pumps suitable for moving liquid have been described and tried.[1] In the early 1950s the most acceptable appeared to be the Sigmamotor pump. A series of bars or "fingers" synchronously and in series compressed the tubing "squeezing" the blood in front of the compressed area (see Figure 9.1). High hemolysis rates and loss of synchronization at high flow rates caused the abandonment of the device, although hundreds of cardiopulmonary bypass procedures were successfully carried out using this type of pump.

The roller pump attributed to DeBakey was patented in 1855 by Porter and Bradley (Patent No. 12,753). Slight modifications have been made through the years, but the basic design is unchanged (see Table 9.1). Today the roller pump is the most common type pump used for routine cardiopulmonary bypass.

A roller pump functions by the rollers rolling along the tubing and compressing it against a semicircular backing plate. As the rollers turn and compress the tubing, fluid is forced in front of the compression area and along the tubing path. A properly adjusted roller pump produces minimal hemolysis (see Chapter 7: TUBING AND CIRCUITS). Even in the early days the pump itself contributed only about 30 mg%/hr to the total free plasma hemoglobin concentration.[2] With more precise roller pumps and better quality tubing this number is probably lower today.

The centrifugal pump entered the present perfusion field in 1972 as an implantable artificial heart. It was not long before they were being applied to routine cardiopulmonary bypass procedures because of purported lower hemolysis rates. The first, BioMedicus, was of a novel design composed of several cones inside a polycarbonate housing. Magnetic coupling of the central cone to an external drive mechanism enables the drive to spin the cones inside the housing. This produces a constrained vortex effect at the circumference which produces positive flow. It is a non-loading pump and flow is directly dependent on the RPM of the cones and the peripheral resistance of the patient.

If the peripheral resistance is elevated, higher RPM are needed to produce the same blood flow rate. If the resistance is reduced and the RPM remains constant, the flow rate increases dramatically. A flow meter is needed to safely perfuse a patient, for without one the perfusionist has no idea what the flow rate to the patient is.

This pump became very popular initially because it was reputed to be air emboli proof. In other words, the pump would not pump air. Unfortunately this simply is not the case.[3,4]

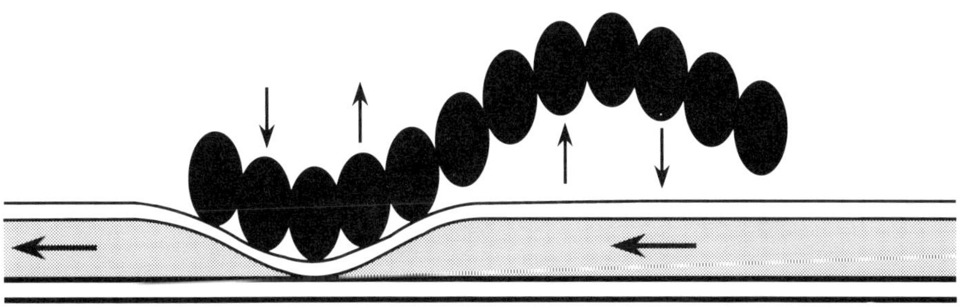

Figure 9.1 Shows the function of the Sigmamotor pump. As the bars or rods vertically compress the pump tubing, blood is forced down the tubing. The bars or rods move up and down synchronously, thus the blood can only travel in one direction.

Table 9.1 List of Patents: Roller Pumps

Patent Holder (Titled)	Patent Number	Date of Patent
R. Porter, J.D. Bradley (Rotary Pump)	12,753	17 April 1855
D. Dieckmann, C. Schmiedtzinsky (Pump)	289,517	4 December 1883
D. Kelly (Rotary Pump)	314,851	31 March 1885
J. Faller (Pump)	328,472	20 October 1885
E.E. Allen (Instrument for the Transfusion of Blood)	365,227	21 June 1987
W.E. Nickerson, A. Berrenberg (Vacuum Pumps)	453,277	2 June 1891
C.H. Truax (Surgical Pump)	459,053	8 September 1891
J.W. Fraser, J.D. Wilson (Vacuum Pump)	496,559	2 May 1893
C.E. Funk (Pump)	513,315	23 January 1894
F.I. DuPont (Pump)	968,599	30 August 1910
M.C. Santiago (Pump)	1,988,337	15 January 1935
M.E. DeBakey, C.E. Schmidt (Surgical Pump)	2,018,998	29 October 1935
E.K. Knott (Pumping Apparatus)	2,314,281	16 March 1943
D.L. Mapson (Pump)	2,332,157	19 October 1943
D. Wittenberg (Rotary Pump)	2,403,572	9 July 1946
H.A. Arnold (Hose Pump)	2,406,485	27 August 1946
L.A. Seyler (Rotary Pump)	2,693,766	9 November 1954
T. Jensen (Fluid Pump)	2,696,173	7 December 1954

*All patents subsequent to Porter and Bradley's are minor modifications on their roller pump prior to its regular use in the cardiopulmonary bypass circuit. This list is not complete.

At a later time it was proposed [during left ventricular assist procedures] that heparinization of the patient was unnecessary when using the constrained vortex pump because clot formation would not occur. This also is untrue (see Figure 9.2).

A more recent version of an earlier centrifugal pump has been marketed by Sarns-3M (see Figure 9.3). Despite appearances the impellers do not seem to add appreciably to the hemolysis rate which is comparable to the constrained vortex pump. This pump is also an non-loading pump and must have a flow sensor attached to determine flow rate. This pump will transmit small air bubbles but becomes locked when presented with a bolus of approximately 40 ml.

Neither pump offers any significant reduction in blood damage during routine cardiopulmonary bypass procedures [less than 3 hours]. The real benefit of the centrifugal pump is in the long term support procedure (see Chapter 22: CIRCULATORY SUPPORT).

All heart-lung machines should be on a routine periodic preventive maintenance schedule. Records of such inspections and any work done on the machine should be kept in the perfusion office. Between inspections, a log book should be kept on each machine and entries made of discrepancies noted during the procedure so that the maintenance personnel can correct the problems. A review of the log book by another perfusionist before using the machine will warn of any potential problems.

Prior to use all functions of the heart-lung machine should be checked (see Chapter 4: CHECKLISTS). The roller occlusions on each pump should be set on each case since the perfusion tubing can vary slightly in internal and external diameter and wall thickness. The pumps should be calibrated periodically, every three to six months depending upon usage. Spare fuses, hand cranks, flashlight, even a spare power cord should be readily at hand.

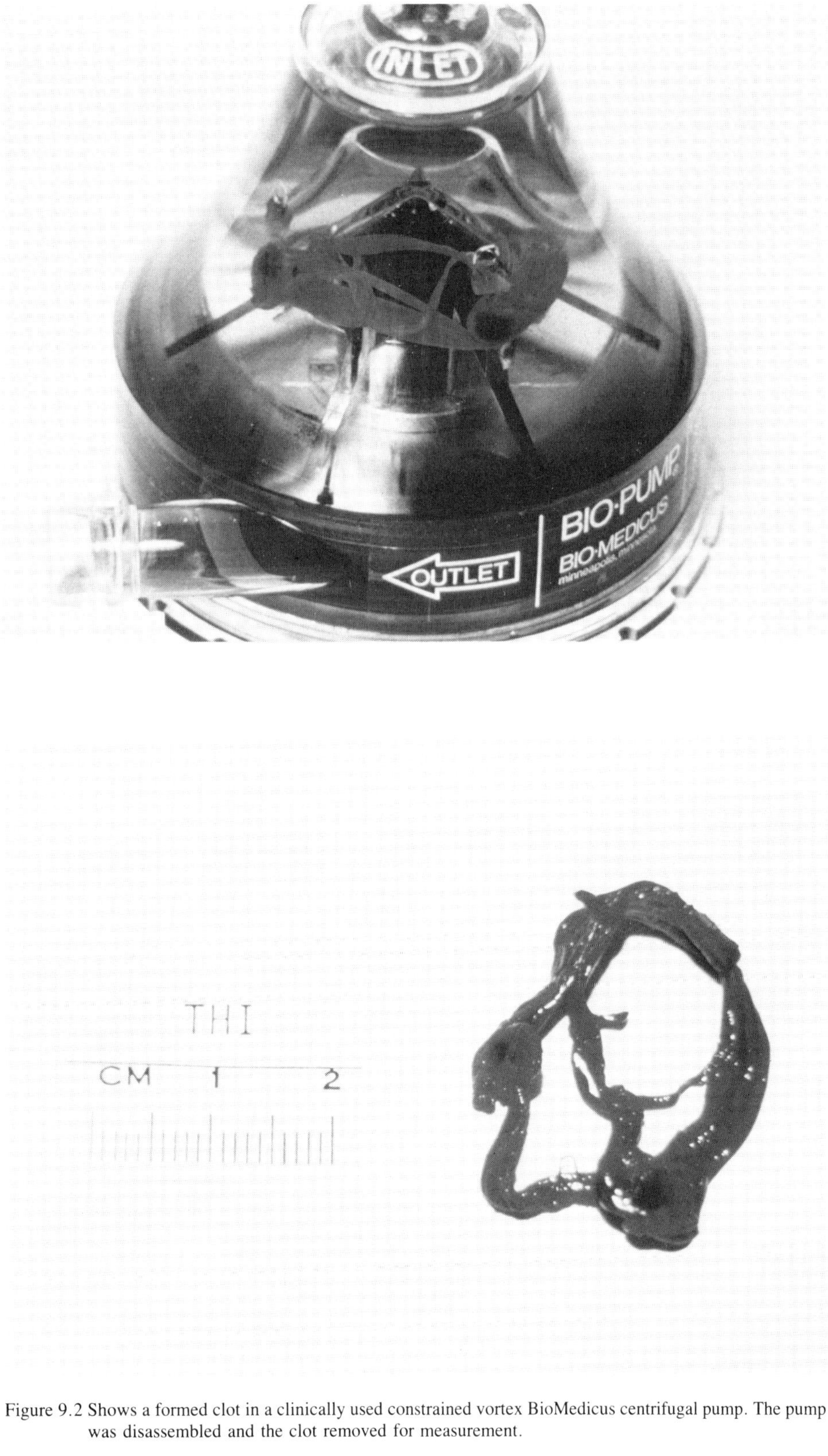

Figure 9.2 Shows a formed clot in a clinically used constrained vortex BioMedicus centrifugal pump. The pump was disassembled and the clot removed for measurement.

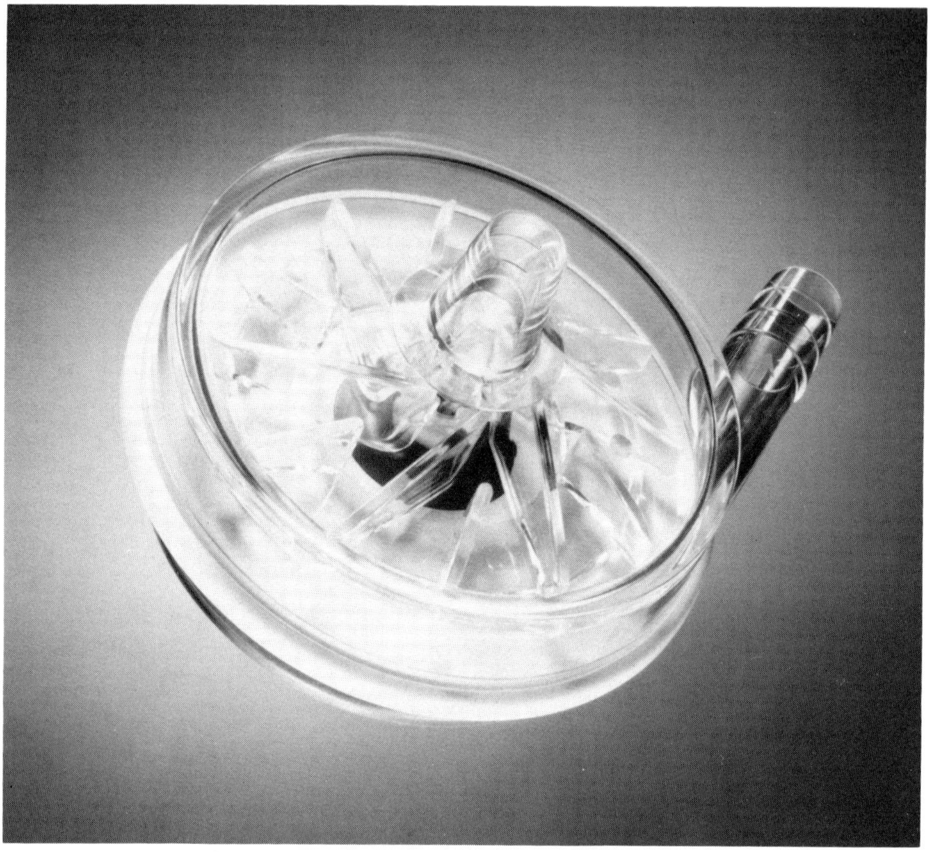

Figure 9.3 The recently available Sarns, Inc. centrifugal pump which incorporates a vaned design.

Jewelry should not be worn on the hands or wrist while working with the heart-lung machine. As with other components of the bypass circuit and with the operative procedure, the perfusionist should be prepared for any emergency which might arise with the heart-lung machine itself. In The Survey, 17% of the responding perfusionists reported life-threatening mechanical failure of the heart-lung machine. There were 335 separate instances reported in the past three years. The accidents included: runaway pumphead, unnoticed rotation of the arterial pumphead, cessation of the roller pump, loss of occlusion, tubing insert failure, reversed arterial pumphead, master breaker burnout, erratic roller pumphead movement, loss of RPM indicator, fire, and bad power cord. The number of injuries and deaths specifically related to these accidents could not be extrapolated from the data.

If more than one pumphead is used and/or more than one operating room is used for cardiopulmonary bypass, uniformity in setup and in the manner the pumps are operated should be observed on all pumps in any room. All pumps should rotate in the same direction on all procedures.

Pumps have speed control knobs to regulate the RPM of the pumphead. The knobs are extensions of rheostats which regulate power to the motor controller which in turn regulates the RPM of the pumphead. The minimum position for the knob stops the pump but it does not turn the pump off. If the adjustment of the minimum position of the rheostat slips or if someone accidentally moves the knob, the pumphead will begin to rotate. This has and can be the cause of arterial air emboli. When the speed control knob is moved to the off or minimum position, the pump on/off switch should be moved to the off position in every instance. Clamping the arterial line distal to the pumphead is an additional safeguard (see Chapter 13: CONDUCT OF PERFUSION).

PULSATILE PERFUSION

The earliest report of pulsatile perfusion was probably that of Hamel in 1889. This was followed by Hooker in 1910 and Gesell in 1913. These studies were concerned with kidney function in the isolated kidney, not total body cardiopulmonary bypass. Since that time reports have periodically flooded the literature as the interest in the technique waxes and wanes. In reviewing the literature the following summaries were obtained.

Normal or pulseless or **non-pulsatile perfusion** has been reported to:

- Alter the pattern of carotid and baroreceptor impulses
- Increase systemic vascular resistance [at low flow rates]
- No effect on systemic vascular resistance [at high flow]
- Alter distribution of blood flow
- Does not alter distribution of blood flow
- Increase lactate and acid production [at low flow]
- Does not affect lactate and acid production [at high flow]
- Decrease oxygen consumption [at low flow]
- No affect on oxygen consumption [at high flow]
- Impair capillary blood flow
- Depress brain function
- Depress heart function
- Depress kidney function
- Reduce lymph formation
- Increase tissue edema
- Produce more histological damage in dog brains
- Increase red cell sludging in dog brains
- Increase perivascular edema in dog brains

During hypothermia it:

- Increases thermal gradients in infants
- Increases cerebral anaerobic metabolism in dogs

During ventricular fibrillation it:

- Reduces myocardial oxygen uptake
- Reduces subendocardial blood flow
- Increases left ventricular compliance
- Decreases postfibrillation ejection fraction

Further, **non-pulsatile perfusion:**

- Does not affect myocardial blood flow
- Does not affect myocardial metabolism
- Does not affect myocardial performance
- Does not decrease renal blood flow
- Does affect renal cortical blood flow
- Does not affect renal cortical blood flow
- Does not affect renal function [at high flow]
- Does reduce sodium excretion
- Does reduce creatinine clearance
- Does reduce urine volume
- Does not affect urine volume

Increases fluid requirements-dogs
Does not effect fluid requirements-monkeys
Increases thoracic duct lymph flow
Increases renin
Increases angiotensin II
Increases antidiuretic hormone
Increases serum amylase
Increases plasma cortisol
Impairs response of the anterior pituitary hormone

On the other hand, reports state that **pulsatile perfusion:**

Decreases peripheral vascular resistance
Does not affect peripheral vascular resistance
Attenuates hormonal changes
Does not attenuate hormonal changes
Increases urinary output
Does not affect urinary output
Increases creatinine clearance
Produces no change in creatinine clearance
Increases lymph flow
Does not affect lymph flow
Produces higher oxygen consumption
Produces no change in oxygen consumption
Lowers mean perfusion pressure
Does not affect catecholamine concentrations
Does not affect glucose tolerance
Does not affect adrenocorticotrophic hormone
Does not affect cortisol
Does not affect rennin
Does not affect aldosterone
Does not affect anitdiuretic hormone
Does affect distribution of blood flow
Does not affect distribution of blood flow

Based on the voluminous literature devoted to answering the question of whether pulsatile or non-pulsatile flow is superior during cardiopulmonary bypass is as meaningful as comparing apples and citrus fruit. One may be comparing apples to oranges or lemons or grapefruit or limes. The problem in attempting a comparative evaluation is extremely complex. A reasonable start would be to clearly define pulsatile perfusion. Until that is done and all investigators comply with that established standard, any evaluations are back to the apples and citrus fruit stage.

The second obvious pitfall is the wide variation in perfusion technique. Many of the differences attributed to the method of pumping are clearly due to the perfusion technique itself. The one important fact that the proponents of pulsatile perfusion have demonstrated is that for normal cardiopulmonary bypass of less than 3 hours duration non-pulsatile blood flow is not detrimental nor does it cause tissue damage.

The controversy is best summarized by Edmunds who stated: "..surgeons must choose whether cost, complexity, and safety considerations of pulsatile bypass are worth dubious and gossamery improvements in capillary blood flow."

These authors do not believe pulsatile perfusion is justified at the present time for routine cardiopulmonary bypass procedures.

An extremely important restriction applies to pulsatile perfusion. Pulsatile perfusion must not be used through microporous membrane oxygenators. The possibility exists that air will be sucked across the microporous membrane during the negative pressure phase of pulsatile perfusion.

REFERENCES

1. Galletti PM and Brecher GA: *Heart Lung Bypass*. New York, Grune & Stratton, 1962.
2. Cahill JJ, Kolff WJ: Hemolysis caused by pumps in extracorporeal circulation. J Appl Physiol 14:1039, 1959.
3. Khoury GF, Mann ME, Porot MJ, Abdul-Rasool IH, Busutth RW: Air embolism associated with veno-veno bypass during orthotopic liver transplantation. Anesthesiol 67:848, 1987.
4. Authors' unpublished personal experiences.

REFERENCES FOR PULSATILE VS NON-PULSATILE PERFUSION

Agishi T, Peirce EC III and Kent BB: A comparison of pulsatile and non-pulsatile pumping for ex vivo renal perfusion. J Surg Res 9:623-634, 1969.

Anabtawi IN, Womack CE and Ellison RG: Thoracic duct lymph flow during pulsatile and non-pulsatile extracorporeal circulation. Ann Thorac Surg 2:38-44, 1966.

Angell James JE, de Burgh Daly M: Comparison of the reflex vasomotor responses to separate and combined stimulation of the carotid sinus and aortic arch baroreceptors by pulsatile and non-pulsatile pressures in the dog. J Physiol 209:257-293, 1970.

Angell James JE: The effects of altering mean pressure pulse pressure and pulse frequency on the impulse activity in baroreceptor fibres from the aortic arch and right subclavian artery in the rabbit. J Physiol 214:65-88, 1971.

Attinger EO: *Pulsatile Blood Flow*. New York, McGraw-Hill, 1964.

Barger AC and Herd JA: Study of renal circulation in the unanesthetized dog with inert gases. (Proceedings of the Third International Congress of Nephrology). Nephrology 1:174, 1966.

Baue AE, Nusbaum M, Anstadt G and Blakemore WS: The pattern of lymphatic flow during extracorporeal circulation. Surg 50:648-657, 1965.

Belzer FO, Ashby BS, Huang JS and Dunphy JE: Etiology of rising perfusion pressure and isolated organ perfusion. Ann Surg 168:382-391, 1968.

Bixler TJ, Magee PG, Flaherty JT, Gardner TJ and Gott VL: Beneficial effects of pulsatile perfusion in the hypertrophied ventricle during ventricular fibrillation. Circulation 60:141-146, 1979.

Black AM: Bicarbonate requirements during hypothermic cardiopulmonary bypass. The relative effects of pulsatile flow. Anaesth Intens Care 4:232-238, 1976.

Boucher JK, Rudy Jr LW and Edmunds Jr LH: Organ blood flow during pulsatile cardiopulmonary bypass. J Appl Physiol 36:86-90, 1974.

Bregman D, Bailin M, Bowman Jr FO, Parodi EN, Haubert SM, Edie RN, Spotnitz HM, Reemtsma K and Malm JR: A pulsatile assist device for use during cardiopulmonary bypass. Ann Thorac Surg 24:574-581, 1977.

Bregman D, Bowman Jr FO, Parodi EN, Haubert SM, Edie RN, Spotnitz HM, Reemtsma K and Malm JR: An improved method of myocardial protection with pulsation during cardiopulmonary bypass. Circulation 56(Suppl 2):157-160, 1977.

Bregman D, Parodi EN, Haubert SM, Szarnicki R, Spotnitz FO, Bowman Jr FO, Reemtsma K and Malm JR: Counterpulsation with a new pulsatile assist device (PAD) in open heart surgery. Med Instrument 10:232-238, 1976.

Chitwood Jr WR, Sink JD, Hill RC and Wechsler AS: The comparative effects of pulsatile and non-pulsatile myocardial perfusion during cardiopulmonary bypass. J Surg Res 30:553-562, 1981.

Chun-Hsiu Y , Bang-Yu C and I-Shan W: Preliminary observations physiological effects of pulsatile cardiopulmonary bypass in animals. Trans Am Soc Artif Intern Organs 27:480-484, 1981.

Ciardullo R, Schaff HV, Flaherty JT and Gott VL: A new method of producing pulsatile flow during cardiopulmonary bypass using a standard roller pump. J Thorac Cardiovasc Surg 72:585-587, 1976.

Ciardullo RC, Schaff HV, Flaherty JT, Donahoo JS and Gott VL: Comparison or regional myocardial blood flow and metabolism distal to a critical coronary stenosis in the fibrillating heart during alternate periods of pulsatile and nonpulsatile perfusion. J Thorac Cardiovasc Surg 75:193-205, 1978.

Clarke CP, Kahn DR, Dufek JH and Sloan H: The effects of non-pulsatile blood flow on canine lungs. Ann Thorac Surg 6:450-457, 1968.

Connolly JE, Wakabayashi A, German JC, Stemmer EA and Serres EJ: Clinical experience with pulsatile left heart bypass without anticoagulation for thoracic aneurysms. J Thorac Cardiovasc Surg 62:568-576, 1971.

Corcoran AC and Page IH: Observations on relation of experimental hypertension to renal clearance and renal ischemia. Am J Physiol 123:43, 1938.(Abstr)

Cowan GSM, Padula RT, Magee JH and Camishion RC: Effects of pulsatile and nonpulsatile blood flow on renal function. Surg Forum 19:389-391, 1968.

Dalton ML, Mosley EL, Woodward KE and Barila TG: The effects of pulsatile flow on renal blood flow during extracorporal circulation. J Surg Res 5:127-133, 1965.

Douglas WW, Ritchie JM and Schaumann W: A study of the effect of the pattern of electrical stimulation of the aortic nerve on the reflex depressor responses. J Physiol 133:232, 1956.

Dunn J, Kirsh MM, Harness J, Carroll M, Straker J and Sloan H: Hemodynamic, metabolic, and hematologic effects of pulsatile cardiopulmonary bypass. J Thorac Cardiovasc Surg 68:138-147, 1974.

Ead HW, Green JH and Neil E: A comparison of the effects of pulsatile and non-pulsatile blood flow through the carotid sinus on the reflexogenic activity of the sinus baroceptors in the cat. J Physiol 118:509-519, 1952.

Edmunds Jr LH and Stephenson LW: Cardiopulmonary bypass for open heart surgery. in *Thoracic and Cardiovascular Surgery* (4th Ed), Glenn WWL, Baue AE, Geha AS, Hammond GL and Laks H (Eds), New York, Appleton-Century-Crofts, 1983, 1091-1106.

Finsterbusch W, Long DM, Sellers RD, Amplatz K and Lillehei CW: Renal arteriography during extracorporeal circulation in dogs with preliminary report upon effects of low molecular weight dextran. J Thorac Cardiovasc Surg 41:252-262, 1961.

Frater RWM, Wakayama S, Oka Y, Becker RM, Desai P, Oyama T and Blaufox MD: Pulsatile cardiopulmonary bypass; Failure to influence hemodynamics or hormones. Circulation 62(Suppl 1):19-25, 1980.

Geha AS, Salaymek MT, Abe T and Baue AE : Effect of pulsatile cardiopulmonary bypass on cerebral metabolism. J Surg Res 12:381-387, 1972.

German JC, Chalmers GS, Hirai J, Mukherjee ND, Wakabayashi A and Connolly JE: Comparison on non-pulsatile and pulsatile extracorporeal circulation on renal tissue perfusion. Chest 61:65-69, 1972.

Gesell RA: On relation of pulse pressure to renal function. Am J Physiol 32:70-93, 1913.

Giron F, Birtwell WC, Soroff HS and Deterling RA: Hemodynamic effects of pulsatile and non-pulsatile flow. Arch Surg 93:802-810, 1966.

Golding LR, Jacobs G, Murakami T, Takatani S, Valdes F, Harasaki H and Nose Y : Chronic non-pulsatile blood flow in an alive, awake animal; 34 days' survival. Trans Am Soc Artif Intern Organs 26:251-255, 1980.

Goodman TA, Gerard DF, Bernstein EF and Dilley RB: The effects of pulseless perfusion on the distribution of renal cortical blood flow and on renin release. Surg 80:31-39, 1976.

Goodyer AVN and Glenn WWL: Relation of arterial pulse pressure to renal function. Am J Physiol 167:689-697, 1951.

Grover FL, Fewel JG, Vinas J, Ghidoni JJ, Arom KV, Norton Jr JB and Trinkle JK: Effects of aortic balloon pumping during cardiopulmonary bypass on myocardial perfusion, metabolism and contractility. Chest 75:37-44, 1979.

Grundmann R, Pitschi H, Berr F and Pichlmaier H: Nonpulsatile versus pulsatile canine kidney perfusion. Surg 75:178-184, 1974.

Habal SM, Weiss MB, Spotnitz HM, Parodi EN, Wolff M, Cannon PJ, Hoffman BF and Malm JR: Effects of pulsatile and non-pulsatile coronary perfusion on performance of the canine left ventricle. J Thorac Cardiovasc Surg 72:742-755, 1976.

Halley MM, Reemtsma K, Creech Jr O: Cerebral blood flow, metabolism, and brain volume in extracorporeal circulation. J Thorac Surg 36:506-518, 1958.

Hamel G: Die Bedeutung des Pulses fur den Blutstrom. Ztschr Biol NSF:474-495, 1889.

Hardung V: Propagation of pulse waves in viscoelastic tubings. in *Handbook of Physiology*, Sec 2, Circulation, vol 1, Hamilton WF and Dow P (Eds), Washington, DC: American Physiology Society, 1962, pp 107-135.

Harken AH: The influence of pulsatile perfusion on oxygen uptake by the isolated canine hind limb. J Thorac Cardiovasc Surg 70:237-241, 1975.

Harris CRS: *The Heart and Vascular System in Ancient Greek Medicine*. Oxford, UK: Clarendon, 1973.

Harvey W: *Circulation of the Blood*. (Edited and translated from Latin by K Franklin), Oxford, UK: Blackwell Scientific Publications, 1958.

Hooker DR: Study of isolated kidney: Influence of pulse pressure on renal function. Am J Physiol 27:24-44, 1910.

Hottenrott CE, Towers B, Kurkji HJ, Maloney JV and Buckberg G: The hazard of ventricular fibrillation in hypertrophied ventricles during cardiopulmonary bypass. J Thorac Cardiovasc Surg 66:742-753, 1973.

Jacobs LA, Klopp EH, Seamone W, Topaz SR and Gott VL: Improved organ function during cardiac bypass with a roller pump to deliver pulsatile flow. J Thorac Cardiovasc Surg 58:703-712, 1969.

Johnston G, Hammill F, Marzec U, Gerard D, Johansen K, Dilley RB and Bernstein EF: Prolonged pulseless perfusion in unanesthetized calves. Arch Surg 111:1225-1230, 1976.

Judson WE and Rausch NH: Effects of acute reduction of renal artery blood pressure on renal hemodynamics and excretion of electrolytes and water. J Lab Clin Med 50:923, 1957. (Abstr)

Kaplitt MJ and Tamari Y: Clinical experience with the Tamari-Kaplitt pulsator: A new device to create pulsatile flow or counterpulsation during open heart surgery. Am J Cardiol 39:260, 1977. (Abstr)

Kohlstaedt KG and Page IH: Liberation of renin by perfusion of kidneys following reduction of pulse pressure. J Exp Med 72:201-216, 1940.

Koushanpour E and McGee JP: Effect of mean pressure on carotid sinus baroceptor response to pulsatile pressure. Am J Physiol 216:599-603, 1969.

Landymore RW, Murphy DA and Kinley E: Does pulsatile flow improve glucose tolerance during extracorporeal circulation? J Cardiovasc Surg 22:239-244, 1981.

Landymore RW, Murphy DA, Kinley CE, Parrott JC, Moffitt EA, Longley WJ and Qirbi AA: Does pulsatile flow influence the incidence of postoperative hypertension? Ann Thorac Surg 28:261-268, 1979.

Lee Jr WH, Krumbaar D, Fonkelsrud EW, Schjeide OA and Maloney Jr JV: Denaturation of plasma proteins as a cause of morbidity and death after intracardiac operations. Surg 50:29-39, 1961.

Levine FH, Philbin DM, Kono K, Cossins CH, Emerson CW, and Austen WG, Buckley MJ: Plasma vasopressin levels in urinary sodium excretion during cardiopulmonary bypass with and without pulsatile flow. Ann Thorac Surg 32:63-67, 1981.

Levine FH, Phillips HR, Carter JE, Philbin DM, Osbakken MD, Boucher CA, Pohost GM, Okada RD and Buckley MJ: The effect of pulsatile perfusion on preservation of left ventricular function after aortocoronary bypass grafting. Circulation 64(Suppl 2) :40-44, 1981.

Levy BI, Bardou A, Touchot B, Menasche P and Piwnica A: Regional blood flow during pulsatile and non-pulsatile cardiopulmonary bypass. Trans Am Soc Artif Intern Organs 27:127-131, 1981.

Litwin MS, Frederick GP, Rubini C, Harken DE and Moore FD: Acidosis and lacticacidemia in extracorporeal circulation: The significance of perfusion flow rate and the relation to preperfusion respiratory alkalosis. Ann Surg 149:188-199, 1959.

Maddoux G, Pappas G, Jenkins M, Battock D, Trow R, Smith Jr SC and Steel P: Effect of pulsatile and non-pulsatile flow during cardiopulmonary bypass on left ventricular ejection fraction early after aortocoronary bypass surgery. Am J Cardiol 37:1000-1006, 1976.

Mandelbaum I, Berry J, Silbert M, Burns WH and Rothe C: Regional blood flow during pulsatile and non-pulsatile perfusion. Arch Surg 91:771-774, 1965.

Many M, Soroff HS, Birtwell WC, Wise HM and Deterling RA: The physiologic role of pulsatile and non-pulsatile blood flow; III. Effects of unilateral renal artery depulsation. Arch Surg 97:917-923, 1968.

Marin MH: Hemostatic mechanisms in extracorporeal circulation. Arch Surg 88:988-998, 1964.

Matsumoto T, Wolferth Jr CC and Perlman MH: Effects of pulsatile and non-pulsatile perfusion upon cerebral and conjunctival microcirculation in dogs. Am Surg 37:61-64, 1971.

Mavroudis C: To pulse or not to pulse. Ann Thorac Surg 25:259-271, 1978.

McDonald DA: *Blood Flow in Arteries*. 2nd Ed, Baltimore: Williams & Wilkins, 1974

McDonald DA: Hemodynamics. Annu Rev Physiol 30:525-556, 1968.

McMaster PD and Parsons RJ: Effect of pulse on spread of substances through tissues. J Exp Med 68:377-400, 1938.

Mendelbaum I and Burns WH: Pulsatile and non-pulsatile blood flow. JAMA 191:121, 1965.

Moores WY, Gago O, Morris JD and Peck CC: Serum and urinary amylase levels following pulsatile and continuous cardiopulmonary bypass. J Thorac Cardiovasc Surg 74:73-76, 1977.

Moores WY, Hannon J P, Crum JD and Willford DS: Continuous and pulsatile extracorporeal coronary perfusion in the beating and fibrillating swine myocardium; Effects on left ventricular function. Surg Forum 28:262-264, 1977.

Moores WY, Hannon JP, Crum J, Willford D, Rodkey WG and Geasling JW: Coronary flow distribution and dynamics during continuous and pulsatile extracorporeal circulation in the pig. Ann Thorac Surg 24:582-590, 1977.

Mori A, Sono J, Nakashima M, Minami K and Okada Y: Application of pulsatile cardiopulmonary bypass for profound hypothermia in cardiac surgery. Japan Circ J 45:315-322, 1981.

Mukherjee ND, Beran AV, Hirai J, Wakabayashi A, Sperling DR, Taylor WF and Connolly JE: In vivo determination of renal tissue oxygenation during pulsatile and nonpulsatile left heart bypass. Ann Thorac Surg 15:354-363, 1973.

Murray WR, Mittra S, Mittra D, Roberts LB and Taylor KM: The amylase-creatinine clearance ratio following cardiopulmonary bypass. J Thorac Cardiovasc Surg 82:248-253, 1981.

Nakayama K, Tamiya T, Yamamoto K, Izumi T, Akimoto S, Hashizume S, Iimori T, Odaka M and Yazawa CF: High amplitude pulsatile pump in extracorporeal circulation with particular reference to hemodynamics. Surg 54:798-809, 1963.

Ninomiya I and Irisawa H: Aortic nervous activities in response to pulsatile and non-pulsatile pressure. Am J Physiol 213:1504-1511, 1967.

Oelert H and Eufe R: Dog kidney function during total left heart bypass with pulsatile and non-pulsatile flow. J Cardiovasc Surg 15:674-678, 1974.

Ogata T, Ida Y, Nonovama A, et al: A comparative study on the effectiveness of pulsatile and non-pulsatile blood flow in extracorporeal circulation. Arch Jpn Chir 29:59, 1960.

Pappas G, Steele PP, Winter D and Paton BC: Pulsatile flow during cardiopulmonary bypass with intra-aortic balloon pumping. Surg Forum 25:134-136, 1974.

Pappas G: A simple method of producing pulsatile flow during clinical cardiopulmonary bypass. Ann Thorac Surg 17:405-406, 1974.

Pappas G: Intrathoracic intra-aortic balloon insertion for pulsatile cardiopulmonary bypass. Arch Surg 109:842-843, 1974.

Paquet KJ: Hemodynamic studies on normothermic perfusion of the isolated pig kidney with pulsatile and non-pulsatile flows. J Cardiovasc Surg 10:45-53, 1969.

Parsons RJ and McMaster PD: Effect of pulse upon formation and flow of lymph. J Exp Med 68:353-376, 1938.

Parsons RJ and McMaster PD: Normal and pathological factors influencing spread of vital dye in connective tissue. J Exp Med 68:869-890, 1938.

Philbin DM, Levine FH, Emerson CW, Coggins CH, Buckley MJ and AustenWG: Plasma vasopressin levels and urinary flow during cardiopulmonary bypass in patients with valvular heart disease; Effect of pulsatile flow. J Thorac Cardiovasc Surg 78:779-783, 1979.

Philbin DM, Levine FH, Kono K, Coggins CH, Moss J, Slater EE and Buckley MJ: Attenuation of the stress response to cardiopulmonary bypass by the addition of pulsatile flow. Circulation 64:808-812, 1981.

Ritter ER: Pressure flow relationships in the kidney: Alleged effects of pulse pressure. Am J Physiol 168:480-489, 1952.

Sachs D, Derry GH, Krumhaar D, Lee Jr WH and Maloney JV: Chemical and hypothermic inhibition of intravascular sludging in extracorporeal circulation. Ann Surg 160:183-188, 1964.

Salerno TA, Henderson M, Keith FM and Charrette EJ: Hypertension after coronary operation; Can it be prevented by pulsatile perfusion? J Thorac Cardiovasc Surg 81:396-399, 1981.

Salerno TA, Shizal HM and Dobell AR: Pulsatile perfusion: Its effects on blood flow distribution in hypertrophied hearts. Ann Thorac Surg 27:539-563, 1979.

Salerno TA, Shizal HM and Dobell ARC: Blood flow with roller vs. pulsatile pump during cardiopulmonary bypass in hypertrophied hearts. Surg Forum 25:141-142, 1974.

Sanderson JM, Wright G and Sims FW: Brain damage in dogs immediately following pulsatile and non-pulsatile blood flows in extracorporeal circulation. Thorax 27:275-286, 1972.

Schaff HV, Ciardullo RC, Flaherty JT, Brawley RK and Gott VL: Regional ischemia distal to a critical coronary stenosis during prolonged fibrillation: Improvement with pulsatile perfusion. Circulation 56(Suppl 1):25-32, 1977.

Selkurt EE: Effects of pulse pressure and mean arterial pressure modification on renal hemodynamics and electrolyte and water excretion. Circulation 4:541-551, 1951.

Senning A, Andres J, Bornstein P, Norberg B and Andersen MN: Renal function during extacorporeal circulation at high and low flow rates: Experimental studies in dogs. Ann Surg 151:63-701, 1960.

Shepard RB and Kirklin JW: Relation of flow to oxygen consumption and other variables during cardiopulmonary bypass. J Thorac Cardiovasc Surg 58:694-702, 1969.

Shepard RC, Simpson DC and Sharp JF: Energy equivalent pressure. Arch Surg 93:730-740, 1966.

Singh RKK, Barratt-Boyes BG and Harris EA: Does pulsatile flow improve perfusion during hypothermic cardiopulmonary bypass? J Thorac Cardiovasc Surg 79:827-832, 1980.

Sink JD, Chitwood Jr WR, Hill RC and Wechsler AS: Comparison on non-pulsatile and pulsatile extracorporeal circulation of renal cortical blood flow. Ann Thorac Surg 29:57-62, 1980.

Spencer MP and Denison Jr AB: Pulsatile blood flow in the vascular system. in *Handbook of Physiology*, Sec 2, Circulation, Vol 2, Hamilton WF and Dow P (Eds), Washington, DC: American Physiology Society, 1963, pp 839-846.

Spickler JW and Kezdi P: Dynamic response characteristics of carotid sinus baroreceptors. Am J Physiol 212:472-476, 1967.

Steed DL, Follette DM, Foglia R and Maloney JV and Buckberg GD: Effects of pulsatile assistance and non-pulsatile flow on subendocardial perfusion during cardiopulmonary bypass. Ann Thorac Surg 26:133-141, 1978.

Taylor KM, Bain WH, Maxted KJ, Hutton MM, McNab WY, Caves PK: Comparative studies of pulsatile and nonpulsatile flow during cardiopulmonary bypass. I. Pulsatile system employed and its hematologic effects. J Thorac Cardiovasc Surg 75:569-573, 1978.

Taylor KM: Pulsatile cardiopulmonary bypass; A review. J Cardiovasc Surg 22:561-568, 1981.

Trank JW and Visscher MB: Carotid sinus baroceptor modification associated with endotoxin shock. J Physiol 202:971, 1962.

Trinkle JK, Helton NE, Wood RC and Bryant LR : Metabolic comparison of a new pulsatile pump and a roller pump for cardiopulmonary bypass. J Thorac Cardiovasc Surg 58:562-569, 1969.

Wakabayashi A, Kubo T, Gilman PK, Zuber WF and Connolly JE: Pulsatile pressure regulated coronary perfusion during ventricular fibrillation. Arch Surg 105:36-41, 1972.

Watkins Jr L, Lucas SK, Gardner TJ, Potter A, Walker WG and Gott VL: Angiotensin II levels during cardiopulmonary bypass; A comparison of pulsatile and nonpulsatile flow. Surg Forum 30:229-230, 1979.

Webber CE and Garnett ES: The relationship between colloid osmotic pressure and plasma proteins during and after cardiopulmonary bypass. J Thorac Cardiovasc Surg 65:234-237, 1973.

Wesolowski SA, Fisher JH and Welch CS: Perfusion of pulmonary circulation by non-pulsatile flow. Surg 33:370-375, 1953.

Wesolowski SA, Sauvage LR and Pinc RD: Extracorporeal circulation: The role of the pulse in maintenance of systemic circulation during heart-lung by-pass. Surg 37:663-682, 1955.

Wilkens H, Regelson W and Hoffmeister FS: The physiologic importance of pulsatile blood flow. N Engl J Med 267:443-446, 1962.

Wright G and Furness A: To pulse or not to pulse, (Correspondence). Ann Thorac Surg 29:489, 1980.

Wright G and Sanderson JM: Brain damage and mortality in dogs following pulsatile and non-pulsatile blood flow in extracorporeal circulation. Thorax 27:738-747, 1972.

..LAWSUITS AND ...CASENOTES

... During cardiopulmonary bypass with a modular type pump a loud thumping noise was heard. The arterial pump was stopped and it was discovered that the blue locking nut had sheared off, permitting the rollers to go to maximum occlusion and remain there. The tubing was switched to the second pumphead and the procedure concluded without incident. The patient was not injured.

... During cardiopulmonary bypass at the point in the operation when the surgeon was suturing in the aortic valve, the arterial pumphead froze. Emergency handcranking was attempted without success. The pump was changed and the patient recovered fully. Examination of the pump later revealed that the drive belt had partially broken and stripped, and that the dangling end had wrapped around the drive shaft of the pulley freezing the pump.

.. The water lines were hooked up in reverse to the heart-lung machine. The patient was cooled and did not respond quickly enough. The water control temperature was lowered more. In actuality the patient was being subjected to uncontrolled hyperthermia and died on the table. The family filed a malpractice suit and the case settled out of court for $1,000,000.

... Six separate reports of BioMedicus pumps that "spew loads of air directly in the arterial side of the circuit."

... During cardiopulmonary bypass the patient suffered moderate hypoxemia which could not be corrected. After bypass and after the operating room emptied, it was discovered that there was a hole in the high pressure gas line from the hospital source that could not be heard due to the other equipment and personnel in the room. The patient made an uneventful recovery.

... Six reports of pumphead tubing rupture due to the design of the pumphead. Examination of the pump revealed that a sharp edge existed on the outflow side of the raceway and that tubing could easily be pinched and cut on that edge.

... During bypass electrical failure was experienced and the perfusionist began handcranking in the wrong direction. Air was sucked into the arterial line and then the perfusionist realized the error and began cranking in the correct direction, pumping the air into the patient. The patient died.

... Two reports of pump-creep. In both instances the patient died. One occurred before bypass began and the second at the termination of bypass. In both instances the alarms had either not been turned on yet or had been turned off at the termination of bypass.

.. Two operating rooms were used and a Sarns 5000 was in one room and a Sarns 7000 in the other room. The 5000 had been modified by the perfusionist in that the forward and reverse switches had been interchanged. In the first room [7000] the vent was run in the counter-clockwise (forward) direction and in the other room [5000] the vent was run in the clockwise (reverse) direction. They had checked the vent under fluid for proper flow direction and occlusion. At the beginning of bypass the perfusionist forgot which room he was in (the 5000 room) and turned the vent on backwards (forward). The surgeon inserted the vent without checking it or without cross-clamping the aorta. Air was pumped into the patient and he died on the operating table. The widow filed suit against the perfusionist, the hospital who employed him, and the surgeon. Plaintiff settled out of court with the hospital and perfusionist for the maximum amount of insurance coverage, $375,000. At trial, in Federal Court, the defendant surgeon won.

... During a hypothermic circulatory arrest period air entered the arterial line, sucked in around the aortic cannula by the negative pressure created by the falling arterial perfusate level. The pumphead was non-occlusive and the arterial perfusate drained back into the oxygenator. The surgeon saw the air and evacuated it before resuming bypass.

... During cardiopulmonary bypass inattention to the reservoir level caused air to be pumped into the patient through the BioMedicus pump. The low level sensor, which was attached and turned on failed to alarm. The patient died.

... Bypass had been completed and the patient was being transfused slowly from the oxygenator. An O.R. nurse passed by the pump with warm blankets which dragged across the arterial pump control and turned it up. Air was pumped into the patient who died the next day.

... Bypass had been completed and transfusion of perfusate in the oxygenator had been completed. The perfusionist stopped the pump by moving the rheostat control nob to minimum. He did not punch stop button. The perfusionist was across the room when a pacemaker lead was thrown across the pump. The lead was dragged up towards the head of the table turning on the pump. Air from the empty arterial reservoir was pumped into the patient. The patient died that evening.

.. During aortocoronary bypass graft surgery the surgeon was performing the distal anastomosis on the circumflex branch of the coronary artery when he occluded the venous return line with his abdomen. Venous return was interrupted and the perfusionist allowed air to be pumped into the arterial line and into the patient who subsequently died. The perfusionist was using a stick-on low level sensor which did not alarm. The perfusionist had twice previously requested the hospital purchase a bubble detector and the request had been denied. There was no preventive maintenance contract on the pump. Suit was filed on behalf of the family against the perfusionist, the hospital, the surgeon who was using a scrub technician as a first and only assistant, and the anesthesiologist who had left the operating room when bypass commenced and was not present when the embolic event occurred. The perfusionist found employment elsewhere. Two weeks after his departure a contract perfusionist repeated the accident with the same equipment, the same personnel, including the absent anesthesiologist, and with the same patient outcome. The case was settled out of court for $650,000.

... The anesthesia department had new O.R. monitors installed and immediately experienced electrical problems in the form of 60 cycle interference. The problem was most pronounced when the heart-lung machine was operating. The anesthesiologists resisted all suggestions from the perfusionists that the heart-lung machines were not defective and that it was a grounding problem or other electrical problem inherent with the new monitors. The problem was easily solved by the anesthesiologists who began the practice of squirting a syringe full of normal saline, D5W, D5RL, or other available liquids directly on the pump tubing within the roller-head raceway. Indeed, this did reduce the electrical interference observed on the monitor screens.

Fortuitously, no patient was on total cardiopulmonary bypass when the pumphead bearings seized, when the motor control units shorted out, or when the arterial line tubing was destroyed from worn bearings which caused the roller-head to oscillate during revolution. All heart-lung machines were repaired by replacing the arterial pumphead bearings and/or drive shafts. The fluid injections were stopped and the monitor problem solved by improving the common ground.

Chapter 10:

BUBBLE OXYGENATORS

Chapter 10: BUBBLE OXYGENATORS

The principle of continuous bubble oxygenation was first proposed by von Schroder in 1882.[1] No experimental survivors were observed until 1950 when Clark, Gollan, and Gupta[2] thought of using silicone compounds as defoaming agents to remove the bubbles introduced in the oxygenator for gas exchange. Until that time, all experiments had ended in failure with the subjects dying from massive gas emboli from the oxygenator. Early open-heart surgery teams built their own oxygenators, e.g., Lillehei, DeWall, Kirklin and Cooley.

Bubble oxygenators were simplistic in design, had few if any moving parts, were easy to manufacture, were disposable, and had low priming volumes. Oxygenation was achieved by introducing gas, usually oxygen or oxygen and a mixture of carbon dioxide, through a dispersion plate directly into the blood. This resulted in a bubble/blood foam mixture in the blood. Early commercial oxygenators used holes punched in plastic tubes or, in one case, holes punched in a plastic disc with old style steel 78 RPM phonograph needles for the dispersion plate. As the phonograph needles became dull the oxygenating characteristics of the device changed appreciably, becoming less efficient. When this was reported to the company by field sales representatives, the company would install new phonograph needles. One oxygenator manufacturer went to the supplier of aerator stones for aquariums and used those for the disperser, referred to these days as sparger plates.

The first commercially available bubble oxygenators were developed simultaneously in Denmark [the Rygg-Kyvsgaard Polystan Oxygenator] and in the United States [the Baxter Laboratories Travenol 3LF Oxygenator]. Both were made by sealing two flat sheets of polyvinyl chloride together either by means of heat or radio frequency welding into the desired design configuration. The Polystan device is still commercially available today.

The evolution of bubble oxygenators was the logical answer to problems of lengthening patient waiting lists, limitations of blood banking, the unsuitability and hazards attendant with utilizing reusable equipment, the need for an oxygenating system that was capable of rapid deployment, and the shortage of trained perfusionists. The bubble oxygenator gained rapid acceptance and by 1972 only a handful of centers in the United States were still using reusable disc oxygenators.

Today bubble oxygenation technology has plateaued. There is very little difference between the various devices available. All available devices generally have venous and arterial temperature ports and luer access ports or manifolds for sampling in the venous line and arterial reservoir. However, they still do not have built-in safety features and devices, and apparently they will not have for reasons unclear to these authors. The next probable development in this area will be that of built-in sensors for electrolyte and blood gas determination and some form of automation of the cardiopulmonary bypass circuit. Specific safety features such as those to prevent massive air embolism apparently will have to wait.

Manufacturers continue today to make small internal changes in the oxygenators without either changing the model number of the devices or notifying the users of these changes. These changes often affect the operating characteristics and it is the reason the authors will not discuss each model available in terms of operating characteristics and parameters. Such information could become obsolete and of interest only from an historical standpoint by the next in-house and unannounced modification.

As stated earlier, bubble oxygenators work by physically bubbling oxygen and other gases directly into blood. They are efficient at the process of oxygenation because they are able to utilize an extremely large exchange surface area, the combined surface area of the gas bubbles, in a very small space, the oxygenating column. If a bubble one ml in size were to be broken up into bubbles 12 microns in diameter, there would be 10^9 bubbles which would have a combined surface area of 4830 cm^2.[3] The oxygenating column on the Polystan for example is only six inches long.

The smaller the bubbles produced for oxygenation, the larger the exchange surface. This has one drawback however: small bubbles are very efficient in exchanging oxygen, but relatively inefficient in exchanging carbon dioxide. The oxygenator must also produce large bubbles to have proper CO_2 exchange. Today's devices produce bubbles in a range of sizes to accomplish both oxygenation and carbon dioxide removal.

A much more significant problem with bubble size in bubble oxygenators is that the more efficient oxygenators produce more gaseous microemboli in the arterial line. In the early 1980s manufacturers moved towards "more efficient oxygenators." Simply stated this meant that with a very low gas flow to blood flow ratio a high arterial pO_2 was produced. At the same time the number of gaseous microemboli produced rose dramatically and in a direct relationship with the "efficiency."[4] The defoamer in the oxygenator is simply not able to efficiently defoam the small bubbles adequately. Gaseous microemboli production detectable in the arterial line is directly related to the arterial pO_2, and inversely related to the arterial reservoir level and the gas-to-blood flow rate. As the gas-to-blood flow ratio goes down and the efficiency goes up, the microemboli count goes up. As the pO_2 goes up the microemboli count goes up. As the arterial reservoir level goes up the microemboli count goes down. These are general observations and, of course, occur within limits and in relationship to each other.

Gaseous microemboli are only removed by defoamer or time.

Regardless of the external appearance of a bubble oxygenator, that is how it looks or what shape it has, internally all bubble oxygenators work in exactly the same way with exactly the same components. These components are composed of essentially the same materials. Figure 10.1 is a schematic representation of the inner workings of all present day bubble oxygenators and a cut-away drawing of a present day oxygenator. Blood from the patient comes by gravity to the oxygenator through the venous line. Blood enters the oxygenator in the area of the sparger plate. Here the blood is mixed with gas and bubbles are formed. The blood is forced upward, in most instances, by the boyancy of the gas bubbles and the upward directed flow of the oxygenating gas.

The foamed blood then cascades downward and enters the defoaming area of the oxygenator where bubbles are removed. This is accomplished when the bubbles encounter a silicone compound, Anti-foam A, and burst due to the reduced surface tension. The Anti-foam A is layered in coats on a substrate which is normally polyurethane foam of a large porosity. In some oxygenators polyurethane filament is used as the substrate.

Secondary oxygenation occurs in the defoaming area. Part of this process is due to the fact that the blood films on the substrate when the bubbles burst and this film is exposed to practically a 100% oxygen atmosphere thus mimicking, in a very small way, the action of the film oxygenators. Another part of the secondary oxygenation is due to the fact that when the bubbles burst smaller bubbles are created momentarily and function within the defoaming area in the same way that bubbles function in the oxygenating area. Since these secondarily created bubbles are much smaller than the original bubbles, oxygenation is much more efficient with these smaller bubbles. Thus the oxygenating efficiency of secondary oxygenation is much greater than that found in the oxygenating column. It has been estimated that 30% to 70% of the total oxygenation takes place in the defoaming area. The exact amount depends upon the oxygenator design. Unfortunately however, the smaller bubbles are much harder to eliminate from the blood for the reasons noted earlier.

If all parameters are held constant during bypass except arterial reservoir level, the arterial pO_2 will vary inversely with the arterial reservoir level. As the level rises, the pO_2

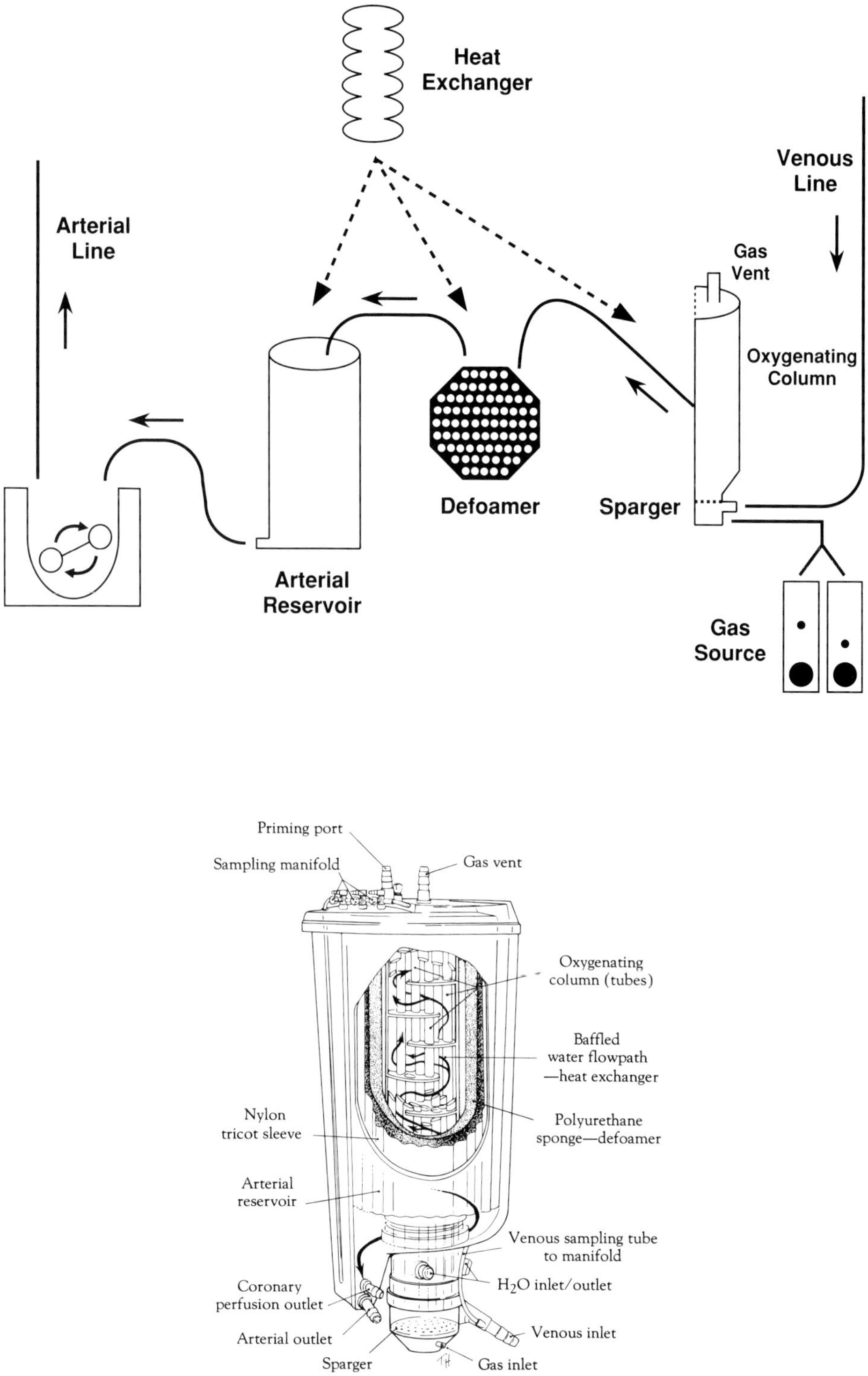

Figure 10.1 at the top shows a schematic drawing of the various components of the generic bubble oxygenator. All components shown are integral to ALL bubble oxygenators. The heat exchanger may be located in or adjacent to all three sections. At the bottom is a cutaway drawing of a currently commercially available bubble oxygenator. Note that all components of the generic oxygenator can be identified in the bottom drawing.

will decrease, as the level falls the pO_2 increases. This is due to the arterial blood rising into or subsiding from the defoaming area, thus reducing or increasing the area of secondary oxygenation.

In order to more efficiently eliminate bubbles from the blood more defoaming silicone compound is needed. Only a specific amount can be applied to a measured amount of substrate. To add more silicone compound to the device more substrate is needed. As more polyurethane foam is added to the device it takes a longer time for the blood to transit the device. As the transit time is lengthened more volume is held up inside the oxygenator. This held up volume has been referred to as dynamic volume hold-up and was used as a sales gimmick at one time, the implication being that less dynamic volume hold-up was better. This is certainly not the case, unless one is totally unconcerned with gaseous microemboli reaching the patient's vascular system.

Thus the perfusionist is faced with the choice of an oxygenating device which is good at removing gaseous microemboli but which requires additional volume due to the hold-up or, alternatively a device in which the blood rapidly transits the oxygenator thus requiring less volume but which emits large amounts of gaseous microemboli. This is, of course, in combination with the size of the oxygenating sparger. A partial list of bubble oxygenators is given as a comparison guide:

EFFECTIVE LARGE HOLE SPARGER, HIGH HOLD UP, SLOW TRANSIT

Polystan Venotherm
Harvey H-1700
Harvey H-1000
Cobe Optiflo II

EFFECTIVE SMALL HOLE SPARGER, LOW HOLD UP, RAPID TRANSIT

Harvey H-1500
Bentley BOS 10-S
Bentley BIO-10
Gambro 10
Shiley S-100
Shiley S100A HED

Another concern to the perfusionist is the question of direct blood-gas interface. Since the oxygenating gas is in direct contact with the blood some deleterious effects occur, the principle one being the denaturation of protein. However, this denaturation effect has also been observed to some degree with membrane oxygenators. In routine open-heart surgery today with current bubble oxygenators these effects are inconsequential. Certainly blood trauma due to the oxygenator is not a question since 90% to 95% of hemolysis occurring during cardiopulmonary bypass occurs in the suction system.[5,6] In those procedures of less than three hours in duration, the bubble oxygenator is a perfectly acceptable oxygenating device that has the added advantage of vast clinical experience.

A polyester fabric surrounds the defoaming sponges and acts as a final gross filter of the oxygenator by inhibiting passage of particles larger than its pore size and which vary with the manufacturer. Normally it is in the range of 100-150 microns. The fabric also aids a little in defoaming, but is ineffective in the very small micro bubble range. In some oxygenators this fabric ends in a gather at the bottom of the defoaming section but some distance above the bottom of the arterial reservoir itself. Care must be taken to debubble under this area since bubbles can be caught in the folds of the fabric. It is also important, during bypass, not to let the arterial blood reservoir level fall below this area since new bubbles may be trapped and subsequently exit the oxygenator due to blood velocity.

After defoaming blood then passes into the arterial reservoir where it is held prior to pumping back into the patient. The arterial reservoir acts as a settling chamber and if blood is allowed to stand in this area, that is to say, a high reservoir level is maintained, the gaseous microemboli count is significantly reduced. A high arterial reservoir level also acts as an additional safety factor (see Chapter 13: CONDUCT OF PERFUSION).

Present day bubble oxygenators have integral heat exchangers to control patient temperature by controlling the temperature of the blood leaving the oxygenator. Except for the Polystan oxygenator, these devices are integral to the arterial reservoir and/or the oxygenating column and defoaming area.

Before use the oxygenator sterile packaging should be inspected and should have no holes, tears or other breach of sterility. After the oxygenator has been removed from the packaging it should be inspected for damage and should be mounted immediately. The gas source should be connected to the oxygenator and the gas is turned on at a rate of no less than 2 L/min to provide a positive pressure on the inside of the device so as to insure that no airborne contamination enters the oxygenator. Appropriate tubing connections can then be made to the bubble oxygenator always using sterile technique.

At this point the integrity of the heat exchange system should be checked. The inlet and outlet water hoses should be connected to the proper outlets and the water source turned on. The water system should be left circulating from this point on. Most leaks occur within minutes, but these authors have seen occasions where the water to blood leak was not obvious for 35 minutes. Automatic shutoff valves and regulators should be checked at this point.

The oxygenator should be mounted on the heart-lung machine in a position where it will always be in the perfusionist's field of vision and where the perfusionist can see the entire device at all times. The oxygenator should be clearly illuminated, and if it is in an area which is poorly lit or in shadow, a light should be set on the floor in a position where the light is shining on the oxygenator. This should be done for two reasons. The first is that most oxygenators today are circular in shape and optical illusions and distortions readily occur in low light conditions. The second reason is that hypothermia is almost universally used now and during rewarming fogging can occur in the oxygenator and again optical distortions can occur in dim light. These distortions can include false readings of where the arterial reservoir level really is.

The oxygenator should be securely mounted in the oxygenator mounting bracket and the integrity of the bracket checked as well as the security of the attachment to the pole on the heart-lung machine.

The oxygenator should be located out of the traffic flow in the operating room, and extreme care should be taken that visitors or operating room personnel **do not go near the device.** The oxygenator should be positioned as low as practical to take advantage of the height differential between the patient and the oxygenator to aid gravity flow. The oxygenator should not be jostled, banged, hit, kicked, or moved during the perfusion. Shaking or mechanical jarring of the oxygenator in any way during bypass will result in an immediate shower of gaseous microemboli out the arterial line.[7] If it is necessary to reduce venous return during bypass, it should be accomplished using tubing clamps, a Hoffman clamp, or mechanical occluding device to partially occlude the venous line (see Chapter 13: CONDUCT OF PERFUSION).

Bubble oxygenators should not be used in cardiopulmonary bypass procedures without a cardiotomy reservoir. The defoamer in the oxygenator simply will not adequately defoam suctioned blood. Secondly, **room air must never be pumped into a bubble oxygenator.** Priming of the oxygenator should be done through the cardiotomy reservoir. The priming solution can be isolated in the cardiotomy reservoir for as long as desired prior to priming the oxygenator and bypass circuit. The arterial and venous lines of appropriate size are connected together with a prebypass filter (see Chapter 8: FILTRATION).

Once priming fluid has been allowed to drain into the oxygenator the entire circuit may be primed. Tapping the oxygenator housing will facilitate debubbling before beginning recirculation. All clamps are removed and the arterial pump turned on at a flow rate of 5 L/min for ten minutes to filter the bypass circuit. During this time the tubing and oxygenator are inspected and all air bubbles removed by gentle percussion.

During a time-critical life-threatening emergency the oxygenator can be primed through the cardiotomy reservoir, the arterial line primed and debubbled, the prebypass and arterial line filtration can be omitted and the venous line can be primed retrograde from the patient. Thousands of bypass procedures have been carried out with no apparent sequelae before the advent of prebypass and arterial line filtration.

Gas blenders must not be used with bubble oxygenators. There is no valid reason to use them and valid reasons not to.[8] The failure rate of blenders is surprisingly high. **Room air must never be introduced into the oxygenator.** The only gases which should be used with the device are oxygen and carbon dioxide. Both of these gases are relatively soluble in the blood stream; thus if an air emboli should occur, the patient has a better chance of absorbing the gas bubble if it is composed of either oxygen or carbon dioxide.[9]

The use of the coronary perfusion outlet should be limited to coronary perfusion which, to these authors' knowledge, has not been used since the early 1970s. Why this hazardous connector remains on bubble oxygenators continues to be a mystery. If a source of blood is needed, for blood cardioplegia for example, a Y connector should be placed in the arterial line and one arm of the Y connector used for the blood source. Y connectors come in almost any configuration and the side arm for blood cardioplegia, or other use, can be purchased in the proper size without further reduction necessary, thus reducing the number of connectors used.

REFERENCES

1. von Schroder W: Uber die Bildungsstatte des Harnstoffs. Arch Exp Path Pharmacol 15: 364-402, 1882.
2. Clark LC, Gollan F, Gupta VB: The oxygenation of blood by gas dispersion. Science 111: 85-87, 1950.
3. Galletti PM and Brecher GA: Bubble oxygenators. Ch 5 in *Heart Lung Bypass*, Grune & Stratton, New York, 1962, p 62.
4. Pearson DT: Gaseous microemboli and bubble oxygenator gas dispersion pore size. Perfusion 2: 227-229, 1987.
5. Keenan RM, Keen WR, Taylor DE, Crane TN, Reed CC: A comparative hemolysis study of bubble oxygenators. AmSECT Proceed 2:39-40, 1974.
6. Keen WR, Reed CC: Iatrogenic hemolysis: A critical study. AmSECT Proceed 3:22, 1975.
7. Patterson RH, Kessler J, Brennan RW, Twichell JB: Ultrasonic detection of microemboli from artificial surfaces: Evidence of microembolic tissue damage. Bull N Y Acad Med 48:452, 1972.
8. Kurusz M, Butler BD: Problems relating to gaseous microemboli and the use of nitrogen with bubble oxygenators. Letter to the editor. JECT 16:113, 1984.
9. Butler BD: Biophysical aspects of gas bubbles in blood. Med Instrument 19:59,1985.

..LAWSUITS AND...CASE NOTES

..Twenty-five minutes into cardiopulmonary bypass for an aortocoronary bypass graft procedure a visitor leaned on the oxygenator or stepped on the arterial line (it was never determined which). The oxygenator fell from the bracket and gas emboli entered the patient. The patient was pronounced dead in the Recovery Room. Suit was filed against the entire team and visitor. The case settled out of court for an undisclosed amount.

... After two-and-a-half hours of bypass the perfusionist noticed an increase in the volume in the bypass circuit. The volume continued to increase over the next 30 minutes when the next blood gas was obtained. The patient's hemoglobin had diminished appreciably. A water to blood leak was diagnosed and the oxygenator changed. All blood was discarded and the circuit refilled with fresh bank blood. The procedure terminated some three hours later. The patient died the following day.

Chapter 11:

MEMBRANE OXYGENATORS

Chapter 11: MEMBRANE OXYGENATORS

The use of membrane oxygenators for cardiopulmonary bypass dates back to the earliest clinical experiences.[1–3] They were touted as "theoretically superior" then, just as they are similarly promoted now. It has only been in recent years, however, that membrane oxygenators have been used extensively for routine bypass. The bubble oxygenator has been used for the vast majority of cases in the past primarily because they are simpler in design and circuitry, cheaper, and have had the benefit of competition among several manufacturers which has led to innumerable refinements in the last two decades. Bubble oxygenators are also simpler to set up and operate.

Membrane oxygenators may be approaching a similar fever pitch of competition, but it is not entirely clear to these authors today that the membrane oxygenator will ever supplant the dominant position currently held by bubble oxygenators. However, this may occur if oxygenator manufacturers do not produce bubble oxygenators which are low in microbubble emission.

Reasons for the failure of membrane oxygenators to achieve their promise have been debated, but no doubt they have been based on no clearly demonstrated clinical benefits to the patient in perfusions of less than 90 to 120 minutes. Certainly papers have been published favoring the membrane oxygenator over bubble oxygenators,[4–7] but others have shown no overwhelmingly superior advantage.[8–12] The Survey asked perfusionists what percentage of their cases they used either a membrane or a bubble oxygenator and it was evenly divided at 50% for either type. The cardiotomy suction and vent systems have remained virtually unchanged since the 1950s, and any small gains in decreased hemolysis due to the oxygenator have been overshadowed by that which occurs during cardiotomy suction. It for these reasons, as well as the lack of conclusive scientific proof that membranes are superior, that makes these authors unwilling to recommend membrane oxygenators for routine bypass procedures of less than 90 to 120 minutes. The authors deplore the scare tactics to attempt to convert open-heart programs to the membrane as a malpractice defense maneuver. There is validity to the use of membrane oxygenators in bypass procedures longer than 120 minutes.

Even though The Survey reported equal usage of membranes and bubble oxygenators, 250 membranes failed during clinical use and had to be changed during bypass and only 107 bubble oxygenators had to be changed under similar circumstances. When asked what type of oxygenator they changed to, almost 30% of the membrane users changed to bubble oxygenators when the membrane failed.

Regardless of the type of membrane oxygenator, they are used and perform in ways different to those of bubble oxygenators. The first fundamental technique consideration when using a membrane oxygenator is that the device must be "sized" to the patient. That is, in general, membrane oxygenators have fixed oxygen transfer rates, and therefore one size will not work effectively on patients of any size. For instance, if a small membrane with a gas transfer rate below that needed by the patient is used, the device will be unable to adequately oxygenate and remove carbon dioxide. If a much larger membrane than is required is used, it will be much more difficult to control blood gases and maintain them in the desired range.

Most membrane oxygenator manufacturers provide instructions as to the rated flow or size of patients in kilograms for the particular models, and these must be followed if one is to avoid being unable to meet the metabolic needs of the patient. These rated flows generally assume a capability of the device to achieve an outlet (arterial) oxygen saturation of greater than 95% when the inlet (venous) oxygen saturation is greater than 60%. It should be noted that even if a membrane has been properly sized, if for some reason such as hypoperfusion or inadequate levels of anesthesia, both of which can drastically increase oxygen consumption, the inlet conditions may fall below the 60% level. This may present decreased oxygen saturation conditions at the outlet, and there can be a period of "catch up" which may last several minutes during which the operating team must attempt to correct the causes of decreased oxygen saturation inlet conditions.

One technique to increase gas transfer in a membrane oxygenator is to recirculate some of the "arterialized" blood. That is a small shunt from the arterial line can be used to redirect blood through the device a second time. Because the inlet (venous) conditions of such recirculated blood is higher than normal venous blood, the resulting pO_2 will be higher than that of desaturated blood that only passes through once. If this technique is used, the total flow to the patient should be compensated for by increasing the pump flow (see Figure 11.1).

The original membrane oxygenators were constructed of multiple layers of thin, solid sheets of material. Blood flow occurred on one side and gas on the other. Carbon dioxide transfer was limited in these early devices because of the reduced driving pressure for that gas and the relative impermeability of the material to carbon dioxide. The spiral coil silicone rubber membrane developed by Kolobow[13] more than 20 years ago has stood the test of time and currently is the only solid or "true" membrane available. Carbon dioxide transfer is adequate with silicone rubber.

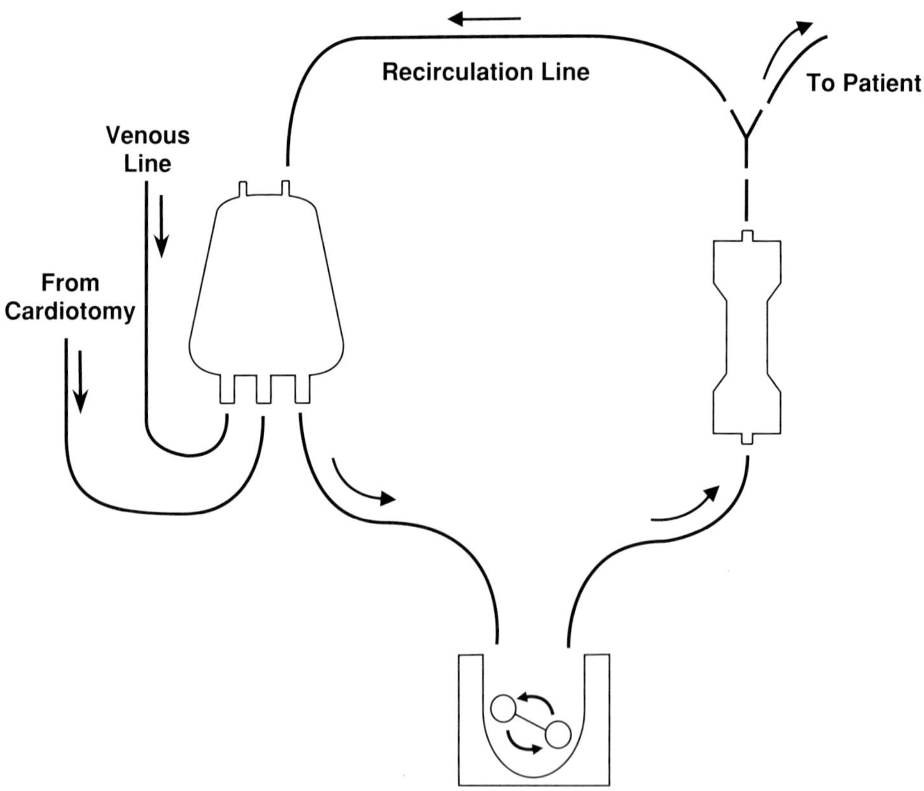

Figure 11.1 Membrane oxygenator circuit with shunt line. Shunt line may be used to redirect blood to increase oxygenation or as an accessory source of blood.

Microporous (polytetrafluorethylene or polypropylene) membranes were introduced in the mid 1970s and have a long track record of use. Because gas transfer occurs across a blood protein layer that bridges the micropores, oxygen and carbon dioxide exchange are excellent. It should be noted that in this regard, gas exchange in the microporous membranes is similar to bubble oxygenators in that there is a direct gas/blood interface, the primary difference being that in the bubble oxygenator it is continually renewed as gas bubbles are formed and broken up.

Most recently, microporous hollow fiber membrane oxygenators have been introduced. The original devices were designed with gas to flow on the outside of a fiber bundle and with blood to flow inside the fibers. Subsequent models work in the opposite way: blood flow is on the outside and gas flow is on the inside. The purported advantage with this design is that if a fiber ruptures blood will fill only one fiber which will not compromise gas exchange. With the former types, if a fiber ruptures, blood will conceivably leak into the entire gas phase possibly compromising gas exchange. Neither type appears to have a particular advantage and both kinds currently are used.

In terms of priming techniques, greater care must be exercised with all membrane oxygenators. A carbon dioxide flush should be used to displace room air. The blood path in a membrane has innumerable folds, crevices and pockets that should be fully wetted to avoid the risk of gas embolism. The carbon dioxide is added to the collapsible venous reservoir bag with closed systems, or it may be flushed retrograde via the arterial filter with either open venous reservoir or closed types (see Figure 11.2 and 11.3).

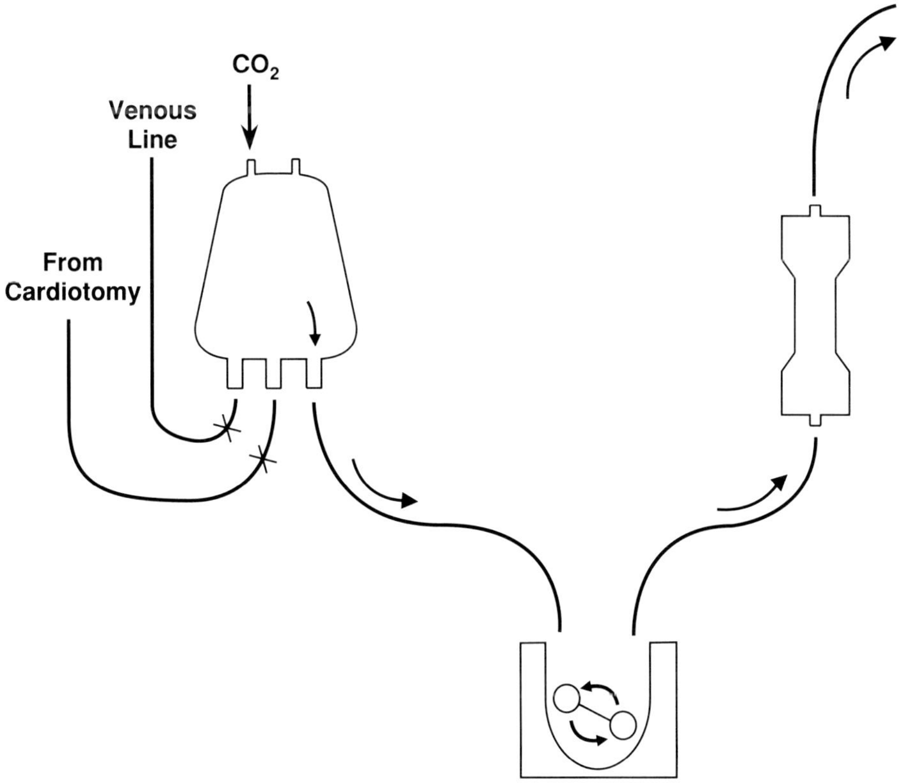

Figure 11.2 Site of CO_2 flush for closed membrane system.

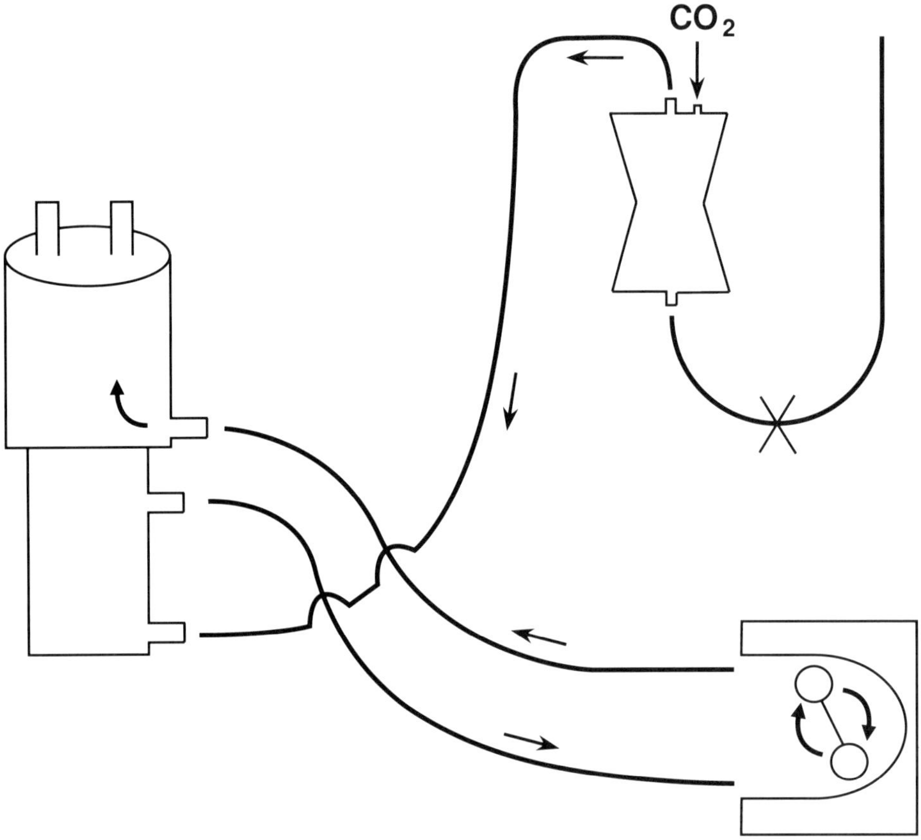

Figure 11.3 CO_2 flush site with open membrane oxygenator retrograde via arterial filter.

If a spiral coil silicone rubber membrane is being primed, applying a vacuum to the gas side in conjunction with a carbon dioxide flush facilitates deairing and wetting. This also has been shown to decrease platelet adhesion.[14]

With microporous membranes, pressure in the gas phase must always remain less than pressure in the blood side, or free gas can be transmitted across the pores where it then can embolize to the patient. This can be prevented by using a "pop-off" valve set to vent the gas flow to atmosphere if the pressure exceeds 5 or 10 mmHg. Membranes may be ventilated with an air/oxygen blender, or, like bubble oxygenators, with two sources of 100% oxygen and 95% oxygen/5% carbon dioxide Yed together. The carbon dioxide levels with a blender are controlled by the sweep rate, conventionally measured as a ratio between the gas flow and blood flow. For example, a blood flow rate of 4 L/min with 6 L/min of sweep gas is 1.5:1 gas-to-blood flow ratio. Oxygenation is controlled in membranes by the percent of oxygen in the sweep gas. The advantage of using an oxygen/air blender with membranes is that it is easy to dial in the desired percent of oxygen. An inline oxygen analyzer, with alarm(s), should be used in the gas line proximal to the membrane any time a blender is used to detect any malfunction of the blender. Membranes also may be vacuum ventilated to avoid the risk of pressurization of the gas phase.[13] However, the use of a pop-off valve would appear to make this technique unnecessary.

It is extremely important that the gas exhaust port of any membrane never be obstructed as pressurization of the gas side would quickly result. Cases of fatal gas embolization accidents occurring when this happened have been reported during routine cardiopulmonary bypass cases and ECMO.

Pulsatile perfusion should not be used with any microporous membrane oxygenator that is placed distal to the arterial pump as gas may be transmitted across the pores if a negative phase of the pulse wave occurs (see Chapter 9: BLOOD PUMPS AND PULSATILE PERFUSION). Advocates of the "closed" membrane system cite less risk of gas embolism in the event that a decrease in venous return is unnoticed by the perfusionist and the arterial pump continues to pump, emptying the bag. With a collapsible bag which contains only blood, the bag will empty, and the tubing between it and the roller pump will collapse and begin "smacking." Gas will be drawn out of solution under these conditions, but massive air embolism is less likely to occur than if an open reservoir is used. It should be noted, however, that using a "closed" membrane system will not in and of itself prevent gas embolism because very little of the gas will go back into solution if the reservoir bag is emptied.

A disadvantage of a "closed" venous reservoir bag is that venous line air must be evacuated periodically. This can be done by either manually aspirating the gas out with a 50 ml syringe or by connecting a monitoring size line to the inlet side of a suction pump. A stopcock should be used to prevent constant purging. Both techniques tend to divert the perfusionist's attention. An advantage of a "closed" venous reservoir, however, is that fluctuations in venous drainage are readily apparent by the distention or collapse of the reservoir bag.

With an "open," or hardshell venous reservoir, venous line air is insignificant because it is dissipated to atmosphere. Most hardshell venous reservoirs also contain defoamer. The disadvantage of a hardshell reservoir is that massive gas can be pumped if the reservoir is depleted. Use of a low level alarm and/or air bubble detector with an open system is necessary in these authors' opinion (see Chapter 26: SAFETY AND SAFEGUARDS).

REFERENCES

1. Bramson ML, Osborn JJ, Main FB, O'Brien MF, Wright JS and Gerbode F: A new disposable membrane oxygenator with integral heat exchange. J Thorac Cardiovasc Surg 50:391, 1965.
2. Clowes Jr GHA, Hopkins AL and Neville WE: An artificial lung dependent upon diffusion of oxygen and carbon dioxide through plastic membranes. J Thorac Surg 32:630, 1956.
3. Effler DB, Kolff WJ, Groves LK and Sones Jr FM: Disposable membrane oxygenator (heart-lung machine) and its use in experimental surgery. J Thorac Surg 32:629, 1956.
4. Boers M, van den Dungen JJAM, Karliczek GF, Brenken U, Homan van der Heide JN and Wildevuur CRH: Two membrane oxygenators and a bubbler; A clinical comparison. Ann Thorac Surg 34:455, 1983.
5. Byrick RJ and Noble WH: Postperfusion lung syndrome. Comparison of Travenol bubble and membrane oxygenators. J Thorac Cardiovasc Surg 76:685, 1978.
6. Dancy CM, Townsend ER, Boylett A, Chan SL, Parker-Williams EJ and Parker DJ: Pulmonary dysfunction associated with cardiopulmonary bypass: A comparison of bubble and membrane oxygenators. Circ 64 (Suppl II):II-54, 1981.
7. Liddicoat JE, Bekassy SM, Beall Jr AC, Glaeser DH and DeBakey ME: Membrane vs bubble oxygenator: Clinical comparison. Ann Surg 181:747, 1975.
8. Edmunds Jr LH, Ellison N, Colman RW, Niewiarowski S, Rao AK, Addonizio Jr VP, Stephenson LW and Edie RN: Platelet function during cardiac operation: Comparison of membrane and bubble oxygenators. J Thorac Cardiovasc Surg 83:805, 1982.
9. Clark RE, Beauchamp RA, Magrath RA, Brooks JD, Ferguson TB and Weldon CS: Comparison of bubble and membrane oxygenators in short and long perfusions. J Thorac Cardiovasc Surg 78:655, 1979.
10. Williams DR, Tyers GFO, Williams EH, Kurusz M, Shaffer CW, Pierce WS and Waldhausen JA: Similarity of clinical and laboratory results obtained with microporous Teflon membrane oxygenator and bubble-film hybrid oxygenator. Ann Thorac Surg 25:30, 1978.
11. Hessel II EA, Johnson DD, Ivey TD and Miller Jr DW: Membrane versus bubble oxygenator for cardiac operations; A prospective randomized study. J Thorac Cardiovasc Surg 80:111, 1980.

12. Hicks GL, Zwart HHJ and DeWall RA: Membrane vs bubble oxygenators; A prospective study of 52 patients. Arch Surg 114:1285, 1979.
13. Kolobow T and Bowman RL: Construction and evaluation of an alveolar membrane artificial heart-lung. Trans Am Soc Artif Intern Org 9:238, 1963.
14. Ward CA, Ruegsegger B, Stanga D and Zingg W: Reduction in platelet adhesion in biomaterials by removal of gas nuclei. Trans Am Soc Artif Intern Org 20:77, 1974.
15. Riley JB and Pfaender LM: Blood oxygenation control by vacuum drawn mixture of room air and oxygen in a membrane oxygenator. JECT 12:40, 1980.

..LAWSUITS AND ...CASENOTES

...The perfusionist decided to use vacuum on the membrane to prime the device. The manufacturer of the membrane oxygenator had designed and installed holes in the body of the oxygenator on the gas side so that it was not possible to accidentally pressurize the gas side by occluding the gas exit port. The perfusionist taped up the holes for vacuum priming. When bypass began an assistant at the operating table stepped backward and in doing so occluded the gas outlet of the oxygenator. The device pressurized and massive gas emboli were pumped into the patient who expired. The perfusionist had forgotten to remove the tape he had placed over the holes for vacuum priming.

...At the start of cardiopulmonary bypass several large bolus of air entered the patient through the arterial line. The patient subsequently expired. Upon investigation it was determined that the exit port for the oxygenating gas had become temporarily occluded which pressurized the gas envelope and it ruptured permitting gas to escape into the blood side of the membrane.

...In an effort to develop a new hard-shell venous reservoir for use with a membrane oxygenator for pediatric cases, a company manufactured several samples of a cylindrical device with an inlet at the top and an outlet at the bottom. The device was used in the research lab before clinical trial with patients. A series of animals were perfused in the usual fashion with the only different device being the venous reservoir. The procedure produced hemolysis manifested by gross hematuria upon institution of bypass. Subsequent tests with the device were done reversing the inlet and outlet. The blood filmed heavily inside the device regardless of the inlet or outlet position used. Further investigation revealed that the device was made from Plexiglas, a known hemolytic material. The hospital returned the remaining samples.

Chapter 12:

MONITORING DURING BYPASS AND INLINE DEVICES

Chapter 12: MONITORING DURING BYPASS AND INLINE DEVICES

Gone are the days of oversized glass mercury and blue-dyed water manometers affixed to wooden boards hung from IV poles. The perfusionist today is confronted with a plethora of devices for monitoring use during cardiopulmonary bypass. These devices range from ones which are absolutely necessary to those that might be termed totally unnecessary. Some in the later category include monitors which duplicate hospital clinical or stat lab functions at an unjustifiable cost to patient care and at dubious reliability.

This chapter contains the monitoring parameters these authors believe essential for performing safe cardiopulmonary bypass. Five specific areas of monitoring are identified: the patient; the venous circuit; the cardiotomy circuit; the arterial circuit including cardioplegia; and other essential parameters.

PATIENT MONITORING

Electrocardiogram

An adequate and reliable electrocardiogram (ECG) must be monitored. The ECG should utilize at least four ECG electrodes to provide the option of changing leads should one become dislodged or broken during the procedure.

Arterial Blood Pressure

An invasive blood pressure must be monitored. This pressure should allow continuous monitoring of systolic, diastolic, and mean patient arterial blood pressure.

Central Venous Pressure

Direct continuous central venous pressure should be monitored. Typical techniques utilize the internal jugular or subclavian vein for insertion of a right atrial catheter.

Urine Output

The patient's urine output must be monitored with a device that permits volume/unit time measurements. Urine produced during bypass should be so noted on the perfusion record.

Temperature

The patient's temperature must be monitored. An adequate and reliable patient site is nasopharyngeal, esophageal, tympanic, or bladder; much less reliable are rectal and skin. Myocardial temperature is sometimes monitored as an assessment of myocardial cooling as an estimate of myocardial protection but is not essential.

Laboratory

A prebypass blood gas, hematocrit, hemoglobin, and potassium analysis is extremely useful, but not essential. The patient's blood gas status must be monitored during cardiopulmonary bypass. Parameters monitored should include pH, pO_2, pCO_2, base excess, and hematocrit. Potassium should be measured prior to starting and stopping bypass.

Electroencephalogram

The patient's EEG should be continuously monitored. A prebypass baseline recording should be available during cardiopulmonary bypass for comparison.

Venous Circuit

There should be continuous intermittent visual monitoring of the venous line and visible parts of the venous circuit during cardiopulmonary bypass. This allows the detection of venous air emboli and possibly clot formation in the venous circuit. Venous inlet temperature should be measured to control cooling and rewarming temperature gradients. A venous blood gas analysis should be performed early during bypass after the application of the aortic cross-clamp.

Cardiotomy Circuit

Continuous, intermittent, visual monitoring of the cardiotomy suction rates should be maintained throughout the bypass procedure. The perfusionist should be alert for clot formation, debris in the suction lines, and excessive negative pressure build-up in the suction line and vent line.

Arterial Circuit

The arterial reservoir and outlet should be continuously monitored throughout cardiopulmonary bypass to insure the integrity of the system, the status of the level of fluid in the reservoir (whether it is stable, rising or falling), the presence of any foam or debris, and general status of the arterial blood volume. The perfusionist's view must be unobstructed and the arterial reservoir must be well-illuminated.

Arterial blood gas analysis should be done *at least* every 15 minutes during cardiopulmonary bypass. The blood analysis should include: pH, pCO_2, pO_2, and hematocrit.

The arterial blood temperature should be monitored.

The arterial line pressure should be continuously monitored. If arterial filtration is used, this pressure should be monitored proximal to the arterial filter.

Arterial blood flow should be measured continuously during cardiopulmonary bypass.

ADDITIONAL ESSENTIAL PARAMETERS

Hundreds of thousands of open-heart procedures have been successfully accomplished on heparin protocol alone. However, a recent survey[1] showed that 97% of the open-heart teams monitored coagulation status. Heparin assay was used by 29% of those reporting and 68% used ACTs. Activated clotting times (ACT) must be measured. A baseline measurement should be obtained prebypass, and the ACT should be repeated as necessary during perfusion to control the values.

The gas flows to oxygenating devices must be monitored continuously during bypass. This includes oxygen that may be added to cardioplegia. If a blender is used, (**only** on a membrane oxygenator), there should be an oxygen analyzer and alarm in the gas line between the blender and the oxygenator.

The temperature of the heater/cooler unit must be continuously monitored during bypass when it is in use.

If the perfusionist is responsible for cardioplegia infusion then all of the items previously mentioned that pertain to the arterial circuit, except intermittent laboratory determinations, should be monitored during the infusion. The laboratory can also determine the potassium level in the cardioplegic solution prior to infusion, a practice which seems logical.

If arterial filtration is used, the purge line and filter should be continuously monitored during bypass to ensure an open purge line at all times and to detect gross air in the arterial filter.

A reliable low level alarm detector should be used on the arterial reservoir. This blood level detector should automatically alarm and preferably turn off the arterial pumphead should this minimum level be breached.

An arterial line bubble detector should be used during bypass and should be installed between the oxygenator reservoir and the arterial pumphead on the negative pressure section of the arterial line.

There are many, many devices available for performing these essential functions during cardiopulmonary bypass, as well as other optional niceties. One must recognize that with the use of any device, essential or non-essential, there is generally an imposed risk to the use of that device. Any perfusionist proposing to use a device for non-essential monitoring during cardiopulmonary bypass must weigh the risk of using that device, as well as the cost, in making the judgment for the efficacy of its use.

Available today are computers incorporated in the heart-lung machine. The computer screens display a variety of information and most are touch-menu driven so that the perfusionist may select, record, modify, analyze, and change many functions during bypass. The imposed risk for use of this novel non-essential device is the distraction of the perfusionist's attention from the arterial blood reservoir level or other essential aspects of the cardiopulmonary bypass procedure.

ADDITIONAL PATIENT MONITORING

Many open-heart teams elect to insert a Swan Ganz catheter for monitoring pulmonary artery pressure. This balloon catheter is floated into the pulmonary artery, and an indirect measurement of the left atrial pressure, or the filling pressure of the left ventricle, is reflected by the diastolic pulmonary artery pressure. Cardiac output may also be measured by thermodilution.

Some centers use direct monitoring of the left atrial pressure through placement of a small catheter in the left atrium. The catheter is then brought through the chest wall and attached to transducers for direct monitoring during and after operation. Air emboli introduced through this system, or sucked into the left atrium around the indwelling cannula will go directly into the arterial system of the patient. Reports of these accidents have appeared from time to time and is the reason this technique is not widely used.

Inline and external devices are available to continuously measure blood gas and/or blood chemistries in the arterial and venous lines of the bypass circuit. Until such time as the inline determinations are economical, reliable, reproducible, and approach 100% correlation with the clinical laboratory, these devices represent an unnecessary and increased expense to patient care. These devices also represent an ongoing unnecessary expense. These authors believe this represents unjustifiable expense unless the clinical setting is such that results of blood gas analyses are delayed more than fifteen minutes, or unless it is in a teaching setting.

Several devices are available to measure the heparin levels in the patient. These tests are considered by some to be useful adjunctive measurements to ACTs. It is the belief of these authors that the bottom line to anticoagulation is the time that it takes a clot to form in a whole blood sample. Therefore, ACTs are recommended as an essential monitoring parameter and other methods are considered adjunctive.

Operating Room Awareness

The final additional monitoring the perfusionist should perform is less specific than the previously described parameters. It may simply be described as operating room awareness. This is particularly important during the pre and postbypass period when the perfusionist should be attuned not only to the status of the patient but also the status of the procedure. The perfusionist is a member of a team of teams and should immediately render any assistance to other team members when necessary. When cardiopulmonary bypass is established the perfusionist's complete attention **must be** directed to the bypass circuit. Secondarily, the perfusionist must be aware of the surgeon's needs in regard to the cardiopulmonary bypass (see Chapter 13: CONDUCT OF PERFUSION).

REFERENCE

1. Kurusz M, Schneider B, Brown JP, Conti VR: Filtration during open-heart surgery: Devices, techniques, opinions and complications. Proceed Am Acad Cardiovasc Perfusion 4:123, 1983.

..LAWSUITS AND ...CASENOTES

.. During cardiopulmonary bypass for aortocoronary bypass graft surgery the perfusionist used an inline blood gas analyzer which displayed digital pO_2. When the perfusionist increased gas flow to the oxygenator the pO_2 increased and when the gas flow was reduced the pO_2 decreased. During bypass no blood samples were sent to the clinical laboratory for verification of accuracy. The operation was completed and the patient was transferred to the recovery room. The patient did not regain consciousness and expired several months later. When the lawsuit was filed it was discovered that there were no recorded blood gas values on the perfusion record or the anesthesia record. There were no blood gas analysis determinations on the patient's chart for the period time the patient was in the operating room, nor were any discovered in the records of the clinical laboratory. The case settled out of court for an undisclosed amount.

...Immediately after the termination of cardiopulmonary bypass the patient's arterial pressure fell. The anesthesiologist instituted pharmacologic therapy. Repeated injections of vasoconstricting drugs produced minimal increases in arterial blood pressure. The surgeon, employing a forefinger manometer, did not agree with the anesthesiologist's clinical evaluation and ordered a sterile monitoring line and needle. The surgeon inserted the needle in the patient's ascending aorta. The ascending aortic systolic pressure measured 245 mmHg.

... The anesthesiologist administered nitroprusside to a patient whose perfusion pressure, measured in the radial artery, was 135 mmHg. The arterial line pressure monitor went from 250 mmHg to 50 mmHg. When the anesthesiologist recalibrated the radial artery pressure transducer, the perfusion pressure was actually 20 mmHg.

... After the termination of cardiopulmonary bypass the anesthesiologist was flushing and recalibrating the transducer which was measuring the left atrial pressure. Air was flushed into the patient. The patient suffered brain damage and subsequently expired.

... The perfusionist was enthusiastically teaching a student during a pediatric cardiopulmonary bypass procedure. While emphasizing a particularly important point, the perfusionist teacher noted a falling arterial reservoir level out of the corner of his eye. He simultaneously stopped the pump and screamed that the venous return had stopped. He then looked toward the table and observed the chief surgeon removing his gown and gloves as he walked toward the O.R. door. There was no patient injury to accompany the perfusionist's embarrassment.

... When instructed by the surgeon, the anesthesia resident administered a full syringe that had been previously filled and labelled "heparin." Baseline ACT was 125 seconds. Three minutes after heparin administration the ACT was 135 seconds. The resident was asked to reconfirm that heparin had been infused. The answer was yes. When asked to show the vial that had been used for heparin, the resident produced an empty protamine vial. The patient was anticoagulated properly and the operation concluded uneventfully.

Chapter13:

CONDUCT OF PERFUSION

Chapter 13: CONDUCT OF PERFUSION

The purpose of total cardiopulmonary is two-fold. The first purpose is to provide the surgeon with a motionless, essentially blood-free and clear operating field by diverting and recycling the scavenged blood. The second purpose is to provide protection of vital organ systems. Cardiopulmonary bypass is not physiologic in any sense of the term, nor can it be physiologic even with membrane oxygenation and pulsatile flow. Cardiopulmonary bypass most nearly reproduces a condition of controlled shock. Present day trained clinical perfusionists may not have heard this comparison, but the same clinical characteristics are apparent. Artificial manipulations such as hypothermia may increase the amount of protection and may increase the length of effective protection. Hemodilution will increase capillary perfusion and flow.

Cardiopulmonary bypass certainly has a basis in human physiology, and other health disciplines, but the predominant influence is clinical experience. This, along with personal bias, fills in the vast void in the knowledge and understanding of total cardiopulmonary bypass. The perfusionist is charged with functioning in this void armed only with the barest of basics in human physiology, rheology, pulmonary physiology, anatomy, pathology, pharmacology, and physics, as well as technological logic. The perfusionist must give thoughtful planning to the ordinary and must expect the extraordinary. He must solve emergent problems logically and deductively and must rely on the experience of the hundreds of thousands of successful bypass procedures which have been performed. The perfusionist must also continue to add to the knowledge base from his personal experiences.

The perfusionist must approach each cardiopulmonary bypass as a separate and distinct procedure simply because the patient is an individual human being who not only deserves individual care and treatment but who also responds in a unique way to anesthesia, the insult of surgery, and to cardiopulmonary bypass. Above all, the perfusionist must keep the safety of the individual patient uppermost in planning for and carrying out cardiopulmonary bypass.

In routine open-heart surgery, the conduct of perfusion begins hours before the start of the actual cardiopulmonary bypass procedure. It begins with the posting of the operating schedule. This schedule orders the perfusionist to begin the conduct of perfusion. The perfusionist must then assemble specific information about the scheduled procedure. The perfusionist must have at hand the scheduled operation, the operating surgeon, the patient's age, weight, height, preexisting pathological conditions, cardiac catheterization data, and time of operation. The second step in the conduct of perfusion is a review of the patient's hospital chart. Most, if not all, information gleaned from the chart review should be recorded on the perfusion record (see Chapter 5: CHARTING).

The third step in the conduct of perfusion is the selection of the disposable equipment and perfusion circuit using existing protocols and the information obtained from step two (see Chapter 7: TUBING AND CIRCUITS).

The next step in the conduct of perfusion is the assembly of the cardiopulmonary bypass circuit. The circuit is assembled in a logical sequence which may vary between two perfusionists or for specific set-ups. For the individual perfusionist, it is important that the sequence be consistent on a day-to-day basis so that assembly of the circuit under urgent or emergency conditions can proceed in a rapid and orderly manner. This automatic response to specific input is only developed by training, repetition, and experience, but will save vital minutes in the emergency situation.

The electrical power and gas supply connections are established first. Next, the various disposables are hung on the heart-lung machine. Once the circuit is assembled the heat exchanger and water source control is tested (see Chapter 10: BUBBLE OXYGENA-

TORS). Next the bypass circuit is primed, preferably through the cardiotomy reservoir system. Many different priming protocols exist adding various and sundry drugs, but all rely on a basic IV fluid for the majority of the prime volume. Normally 20 ml/kg is the factor used to determine priming volume. If less is used, the perfusionist will find that, during the bypass, he will be translocating volume from the patient to the oxygenator to maintain a safe reservoir level. This will have an adverse effect on the perfusion pressure. It is better to prime with at least 20 ml/kg and avoid the subsequent problems.

The circuit is recirculated, debubbled, and filtered. The prebypass filter is removed, the pump occlusions set and the lines affixed to the operative field. Alternatively the lines are received from the operative field and connected to the corresponding pump-side lines. The arterial and venous lines should be clamped at the pump and controlled by the perfusionist. When the pump is shut off the perfusionist should clamp the arterial and venous lines at the pump and control those clamps even if the surgeon also clamps the lines at the operating table. Surgeons should be supplied regular tubing clamps and should not substitute other surgical clamps because they will not adequately occlude PVC tubing. All eight-inch clamps should be barred from the operating room. This size clamp will not occlude smaller size tubing and, in some instances, will not even occlude half-inch tubing. Accidents have been reported where lines were not occluded and air traveled to the operative field or blood drained from the operative field partially exsanguinating the patient.

At this point the system should be ready to commence bypass, the checklist should have been completed (see Chapter 4: CHECKLISTS), the perfusion record should have been completed to this stage, and the perfusionist should be ready to start cardiopulmonary bypass. The perfusionist should be aware of the stage of the operation at all times during set-up and should be prepared to start cardiopulmonary bypass at any time should an emergency arise. It is advisable to have a full liter bag of priming solution connected to the quick prime port of the cardiotomy reservoir before starting cardiopulmonary bypass. This practice could save minutes later in an emergency need for fluid volume.

In most open-heart programs the anesthesiologist will administer the calculated heparin dose when the surgeon begins to cannulate the heart, although some surgeons still inject the heparin directly into the right atrium themselves. These authors believe that it is the responsibility of the perfusionist to verbally verify the administration of the initial heparin dose. This serves as a safety check so that the heparin is not inadvertently forgotten and cannulation completed and bypass begun with no heparin in the patient — a complication which has been reported on more than one occasion. The heparin effect may be measured by ACT three to five minutes after injection of the drug.

Those alarms and sensors which can be turned on and activated at this point in the procedure should be turned on and activated. All other alarms should be turned on and activated as soon as possible after bypass has begun.

The technique of "sequestration" is still used by some open-heart teams on routine cardiopulmonary bypass procedures. This entails draining up to 1500 ml or more of the patient's blood into a holding reservoir and replacing it in the patient with an equal volume of electrolyte fluid. This is a bad technique and should no longer be used for routine open-heart surgery. The first glaring fallacy in the technique is the volume-for-volume replacement. It has been clearly established that up to seven volumes of electrolyte for one volume of blood removed are needed to adequately re-equilibrate the hemodynamics.[1] The second fallacy is that electrolyte solution does not contain 2,3-DPG, thus it may transport oxygen in solution but does not transfer that oxygen. The authors have witnessed polycythemic pediatric patients destabilize hemodynamically and cardiopulmonary bypass started on an emergency basis due to using this technique. The same result can occur in the adult polycythemic patient. The third fallacy is that the cardiopulmonary bypass circuit does not destroy formed elements of the blood as it once did, thus the benefit of the saving of "good" blood is not significant. The fourth problem is the metabolic alkalosis resultant from massive electrolyte infusion. The technique may have had some small merit in the 1960s, but has no place in today's cardiopulmonary bypass techniques.

Specific fluid selection for priming also differs from team to team. These authors believe that the preferable priming solution is 5% dextrose in lactated Ringer's solution, although some of the premixed solutions have merit. Priming solutions without glucose should be avoided vigorously. A recent study showed that patients in which only lactated Ringer's solution was used required almost ten times as much supplementary fluid during bypass than patients in which 5% dextrose in lactated Ringer's solution was used in order to maintain adequate flow rates.[2] Adequate flow rates were defined as 50 ml/kg/min. The use of normal saline or 5% dextrose in water as a priming solution is even a worse choice and presents more profound supplemental fluid requirements and problems.

When instructed by the surgeon to start bypass, the perfusionist should release the arterial line clamp, then place the arterial pumphead in the forward mode direction, and then release the venous line clamp.

The perfusionist should watch the arterial line pressure monitor as he slowly increases arterial flow. If no arterial line pressure monitor is available the perfusionist should hold and slightly squeeze the arterial line as the arterial flow is increased. A sudden rise in arterial line pressure or a sudden hardening of the arterial line may well indicate a dissection somewhere in the patient's arterial system. The perfusionist should *immediately stop the pump* and clamp the venous line and then clamp the arterial line while simultaneously notifying the operating surgeon of the perfusionist's actions and suspected condition in the patient. Even if later proved wrong, the perfusionist should initiate and carry out these actions rapidly and independently if the indications are present. Arterial dissections are abrupt, rapid, and frequently fatal, while almost all bypass procedures may be safely stopped momentarily at this stage of the operation. If dissection is even remotely suspected it is better to be wrong in your actions than wrong in not acting. The patient's life may depend upon the decisiveness of the perfusionist at this critical time in the procedure.

The arterial filter purge line must be opened at this time to ensure a constant low pressure vent for gaseous microemboli or massive air emboli.

At the start of cardiopulmonary bypass the arterial pressure will drop precipitously and may continue in this hypotensive state for a period of time. This is the direct result of rapid and severe hemodilution and the change in viscosity of the patient's blood with the resultant change in peripheral resistance. The effect is usually transitory. Administration of vasoconstrictive drugs can artificially overcome this effect. The perfusionist can partially compensate for the hypotension by starting the arterial pump slowly before removing the venous clamp. Then, when adequate arterial flow is established, the perfusionist can partially occlude the venous line, translocating blood into the venous system of the patient. The limiting factor is the availability of blood volume which, of course, varies from patient to patient. Enough volume must be maintained in the arterial reservoir to provide a safe operating level. There comes a point where any action on the part of the perfusionist to compensate for the hemodilution effects becomes ineffective. **The perfusionist can only pump to the operating table the fluid volume which comes from the operating table.** Arterial flow can only be increased so much, venous return can only be retarded so much. Beyond that point the perfusionist is incapable of further effective action.

If single atrial cannulation is being employed, there is little the perfusionist can do to overcome this hypotensive effect. If the venous line is partially clamped, the operating field or the anastomosis site will be flooded with blood. The possibility of pulmonary congestion and edema also exist during such compensatory maneuvers. A greater risk is the potentially lethal overdistension of the left heart if venting is inadequate or not used when the heart is not beating.

The current thinking about perfusion pressure seems to be that either 35 mmHg and higher is acceptable or that higher pressure (greater than 50 mmHg) is mandatory, thus the hypotension at the start of bypass and its possible continuation presents cause for concern to some. Many teams are grappling with this problem which is exacerbated with single atrial cannulation. The only solution available appears to be administration of a vasoconstrictive drug which artificially increases peripheral resistance and constricts most vascular beds. This action would reduce capillary perfusion and slightly increase blood volume requirements by increasing circulation time. This seems diametrically opposed to what perfusion is about. The use of pulsatile perfusion further potentiates the problem since it further reduces peripheral vascular resistance, thus reducing the perfusion pressure additionally.

VENOUS RETURN

Venous return to the oxygenator is by gravity, and the height differential between the right atrium of the patient and the oxygenator should be employed to the maximum optimal effect. Beyond this point the venous return may decrease due to the almost complete drainage of the venous circulation and the resultant collapse of the venous vasculature.

Having exceeded the maximum allowable gravity force is sometimes diagnosed by a continuous or intermittent popping or jerking of the venous line. If the central venous pressure is being monitored by transducer a phasic rise and fall in pressure may be observed. At other times a reduced venous return is the only observable factor. Raising the oxygenator should correct the problem. If the venous return increases when the oxygenator is raised there was too much height differential for the blood volume available.

If the venous return is lower than anticipated, the perfusionist should first lower the oxygenator. If lowering the oxygenator does not improve the venous return then the oxygenator should be raised. If this maneuver does not improve venous return the perfusionist should inform the surgeon and ask that the cannulae be checked for malposition. The surgeon may assist by raising the operating table if no malposition is discovered. The anesthesiologist can also assist by inspecting the patient's head, neck, and upper extremities. If venous return is still low, and no other problem is detected, the physician(s) may prescribe the addition of fluids to the bypass circuit if protocol does not address this problem.

Venous return with a closed membrane system is limited by the volume capacity of the venous reservoir bag and height of the excess fluid in the cardiotomy reservoir in relation to the height of the patient's heart. Regulating the height of the cardiotomy reservoir will increase or decrease venous return with a closed membrane system.

CARDIOTOMY SUCTION

The cardiotomy suckers **must never** be turned on until the heparin has been administered. The perfusionist must check with the anesthesiologist to ensure that the heparin has been given. In some teams the anesthesiologist automatically announces this to the perfusionist and the surgeon. Some perfusionists record the time and amount of heparin administration on the perfusion record, even though this is being recorded on the anesthesia record, and this is a practice the authors endorse.

The cardiotomy suckers should be operated at a speed that ensures adequate blood clearance at the operative field. They should be operated no faster than necessary. It was DeWall who stated, "Unfortunately many surgeons use the cardiotomy suction as though it were the bilge pump on the Andrea Doria."[6] When not in use, the suckers should be turned off. This will reduce the percolating effect in the cardiotomy suction system. Another way to reduce this percolating effect is to lower the cardiotomy reservoir to or near the level of the suction pumpheads. This may slow drainage from the cardiotomy reservoir, but on 90-95% of the open-heart cases this is of little or no consequence.

The suckers must be turned off prior to the administration of protamine. Protamine should never be administered through the pump system. There is some controversy in stopping the suckers this early. The argument against this practice is that the protamine takes three to five minutes to circulate effectively. The authors would urge review of a study which indicated how rapidly fat was detected in the right atrium from dividing the sternum.[3] If ordered to leave the pump suctions on after the administration of protamine, it is the responsibility of the perfusionist to protect as much of the perfusion circuit as possible in the event that blood clotting occurs in the bypass circuit. Clamping the cardiotomy return line to the oxygenator just distal to the reservoir or between the reservoir and the extracorporeal filter if one is in use will accomplish this. If clotting occurs and cardiopulmonary bypass must be restarted, the oxygenator and arterial and venous line should be clot free using this procedure. The perfusionist will then only need to change out the clotted cardiotomy reservoir to have a relatively safe system.

VENT

The vent line **must** be checked for flow direction prior to insertion into the heart. This is most easily accomplished by one of the surgeons dipping the vent in some physiological fluid at the operative field and verifying that the vent is sucking instead of blowing air. There is usually a little fluid in the pericardial bowl and sticking the sucker into that will show whether the vent is blowing bubbles or aspirating fluid. The perfusionist **must** check the tubing direction through the pumphead, the pumphead rotation direction, and the occlusion of the pumphead just prior to use by the surgeon. The safest set-up for the vent line is one in which a 25 gauge needle is inserted in the vent line about 6-8 inches proximal to the vent itself. This acts as a suction relief and prohibits excessive negative pressure from building up in the line. There are commercially available one-way valves which do the same thing. In those situations where the surgeon does not use a vented vent line or pressure relief valve, the perfusionist must pay greater attention to the vent pump operation. When the tubing is observed to be collapsed or a "smacking" sound is heard, the vent pump should be stopped. Suction will still be exerted in the vent line as long as the tubing is collapsed. When the obstruction at the vent tip is relieved, the pumphead tubing will rebound and normal operation of the vent pump can be resumed.

Use of one-way valves of the duck-bill type are in opposition to the philosophy of a large bore sucker and vent tubing because the orifice through the duck-bill portion is very small. Use of a one-way valve is the best choice from a malpractice stand point. However, there have been reports of these valves being inserted in the vent line backwards.

Venting during cardioplegia infusion is ineffective, but causes no more problems or presents no more hazards than has been listed (see Chapter 25: AIR).

CARDIOTOMY RESERVOIR

The cardiotomy reservoir is a device in which blood may be temporarily stored, and salvaged blood may be filtered and defoamed prior to being returned to the oxygenator. An oxygenator is not designed or manufactured to adequately defoam the froth, scud, blood, and room air which are recovered through the suction and vent system. Letting the suction blood directly transit the cardiotomy reservoir and return to the oxygenator is an extremely poor technique because the gaseous microemboli count in the arterial line will be much higher if this technique is used and the size of the bubbles also will increase.

The correct use of the cardiotomy reservoir is to accumulate suctioned blood until 100 to 300 ml or more of blood is recovered, and then unclamp the cardiotomy return line and let this blood drain into the oxygenator. Increasing the dwell time in the reservoir will assist adequate defoaming of the suction blood, and the longer the dwell time the better the debubbling. In using a bubble oxygenator one might retort that the suctioned blood is defoamed, let into the oxygenator, and simply foamed again. This is only partially true. Importantly, the bubbling in the oxygenator produces oxygen and perhaps carbon dioxide bubbles of a specific size range, while the suction system produces air bubbles and foam of a wide range of sizes, and it is the small end of the spectrum which is poorly handled by the oxygenator. Bubbles composed of O_2 and CO_2 resolve faster than air bubbles due to the solubility differences, and are tolerated at the tissue level far better than those containing nitrogen (see Chapter 26: AIR). Proper use of the cardiotomy reservoir will appreciably reduce the microemboli emission through the arterial line.

DURING BYPASS

During cardiopulmonary bypass the perfusionist should monitor all aspects of the perfusion circuit, the physiological patient monitors, the operating team, the anesthesiologist, as well as traffic near the pump. This monitoring should be done on a continual orderly scanning basis. The attention of the perfusionist should not become fixed on any one aspect of the perfusion for longer than two or three seconds. Nothing should be allowed to break this train of scanning observation.

A relaxed atmosphere in the operating room is certainly desirable since the various teams respond better to additional transient stress occurrences in such a setting. On principle, however, communication during bypass should be limited to that which only concerns the patient on bypass. All such communication directed to the perfusionist should be acknowledged by the perfusionist to avoid either misunderstanding what was said or not hearing what was said. The perfusionist should communicate to the surgeon any abnormal observations such as abrupt and/or sustained decreases in venous return or increases in arterial line pressure or other deviations from a normal bypass.

During cardiopulmonary bypass the perfusionist should make record entries whenever one of the perfusion parameters is changed or changes. An entry should be made at least every fifteen minutes even without a change in any of the perfusion parameters. Perfusion parameters include: arterial flow rate, gas flow rate(s), perfusion pressure, patient temperature, and blood gas analysis. When an entry is made every blank on the perfusion record should be filled in (see Chapter 5: CHARTING).

A blood gas analysis should be obtained approximately 5 to 10 minutes after the start of bypass. Another should be drawn five minutes after the aortic cross-clamp has been applied or if any partial bypass has continued longer than fifteen minutes. This first blood gas drawn on total bypass will give an analysis of oxygenator performance and hemodilution effects. If that value is within the normal range then the analysis should be repeated in 30 minutes if all other perfusion and patient parameters remain the same. If any perfusion parameter is changed then the blood gas analysis should be repeated. A blood gas analysis should be drawn just prior to termination of bypass.

The perfusionist should attempt to keep the blood gas values at pH 7.40, pCO_2 40 mmHg, pO_2 between 100 and 200 mmHg, K^+ 4.0 mEq/L. These are the desired values at normothermia and uncorrected hypothermia. Hypothermia values should be reported to the perfusionist uncorrected and measured at 37° C. Contrary to the published opinion of some investigators, the two separate gas values can be controlled by the perfusionist using bubble oxygenators. The use of two gas sources, one of 100% O_2 and one of 5% CO_2-95% O_2, will allow the manipulation of each gas partial pressure independently.

If the pO_2 is increased from 230 mmHg to 340 mmHg, holding the flow rate, the arterial reservoir level, and all other parameters constant, there will be a six-fold, or 600%, increase in the gaseous microemboli count of bubbles > 50 microns in size in the arterial line.[4]

Continual evaluation of the coagulation status of the patient on cardiopulmonary bypass should be available to the perfusionist. This is usually in the form of ACTs. The Survey reports that 68% of the responding perfusionists have observed clots in components of the cardiopulmonary bypass circuit which represented 388 cases with four injuries and 27 deaths in a three year period of time.

During cardiopulmonary bypass the perfusionist should maintain an operating level in the arterial reservoir equal to **at least 25% of the arterial blood flow.** This should give the perfusionist at least a 15 second safety margin should venous return be abruptly interrupted. An even higher operating level is advisable if the blood volume is available and the patient's condition allows it. To operate the oxygenator with a lower blood level is to invite disaster in the form of perfusion accidents. Lower operating levels will also increase production and transmission of gaseous microemboli. Lower operating levels simply cannot be justified today with the wide range of perfusion equipment available. The oxygenator should be operated with the reservoir level higher than the manufacturer's recommendation, in fact the higher the better.[4]

When bypass is terminated the heart will either contract effectively or it will not contract effectively. If the heart fails to eject effectively it may be supported using the heart-lung machine and partial bypass. Partial bypass should not be prolonged. During partial cardiopulmonary bypass the perfusionist really has no idea about the total perfusion flow to the patient. He only knows about that part of the flow originating from the heart-lung machine. Additionally, the arterial blood pressure is usually not treated as vigorously since the patient is being partially supported by the heart-lung machine and much lower pressures have been tolerated during the cardiopulmonary bypass procedure. The patient must be ventilated during any partial bypass situation.

During partial cardiopulmonary bypass the blood gases are not usually adequately monitored and appropriate corrections are often overlooked due to the belief that bypass will be ending shortly. Time can pass quickly and the normothermic patient can be irreparably harmed by unrecognized hypoperfusion and/or inadequate oxygenation. The goal should be to start and terminate cardiopulmonary bypass as rapidly as is safely possible. Partial bypass is not an innocuous technique and has proved injurious and even fatal. Should circulatory support be needed for the failing heart, proper procedures (IABP or LVA) can and should be instituted according to circumstances (see Chapter 22: CIRCULATORY SUPPORT).

At the termination of cardiopulmonary bypass the perfusionist should clamp the venous line at the pump and reduce arterial flow in a smooth coordinated manner. Extreme caution must be observed at this time so that the left heart is not overfilled. Good communication is essential at this point in the procedure between the surgeon and/or anesthesiologist who are directly observing the heart and the perfusionist whose observations are limited to the patient monitor and arterial blood reservoir. Importantly, the anesthesiologist must be aware that the patient is now functioning independent of the heart-lung machine. Cases of the anesthesiologist "forgetting" to resume lung ventilation have occurred in the immediate postbypass period. Distending the heart may cause irreversible damage to the myocardium. Transfusion of the contents of the arterial reservoir should continue within protocol or on prescription. When no more blood is needed the pump should be turned off with the switch, not just with the rheostat control knob.

Transfusion of blood through the aortic cannula is hazardous. It is a utilized technique in spite of continued reports of gross air emboli being infused during this procedure. Alternatives are available to the open-heart team. The most direct is to transfuse the patient from the pump into a peripheral or internal jugular vein or directly into the right atrium. The second is to pump the oxygenator contents into IV bags and drip infuse through the same sites.

A novel technique has been recently described which reduces the chance of arterial air emboli and reduces the chance of over-distention of the heart. This technique involves a shunt line or AV loop between the arterial and venous line. At the termination of bypass the shunt is opened and the arterial line clamped. Blood is then transfused into the right heart.[5] This technique is not without hazard however. If the clamps on the shunt between the venous and arterial line are not completely occlusive, (and the shunt line should be double clamped), air can be drawn from the venous line across the shunt and pumped into the patient through the arterial line. This will occur distal to any air bubble detector or arterial line filter protection.

Once the bypass has been terminated, the arterial reservoir level should not be transfused below the bottom of the defoamer in most bubble oxygenators until the open-heart team is relatively certain that bypass will not be reinstituted. The reason for this is that air bubbles can become trapped in the folds of the defoamer if the arterial reservoir level is permitted to rise again. These bubbles may be swept into the arterial line if full flow is reestablished. Completely emptying a membrane oxygenator presents the perfusionist with the same problems.

POSTBYPASS

The perfusionist's responsibilities to the patient do not end as soon as cardiopulmonary bypass is terminated. The perfusionist should continue to monitor the patient's hemodynamics and be prepared to restart bypass at the surgeon's direction. The perfusionist should not begin disassembly of the circuit until after the surgeon passes off the pump lines. In the case of the unstable patient, disassembly of the bypass circuit should be delayed until the sternal wires are in place.

The immediate postbypass period seems to be a particularly vulnerable time for the open-heart patient. These authors have enough collective intelligence to not enter the "protamine reaction" controversy which has raged back and forth across the head of the table and which has remained unresolved for so long. However, information was obtained from The Survey which emphasizes the hazards of this period of the open-heart operation. In response to a question concerning a "protamine reaction" 72% of the respondents indicated they had observed such an occurrence. These authors are convinced that the perfusionists were not diagnosing a clinical event or making a clinical judgment but rather echoing what they were hearing and observing and which originated from the surgeon and/or anesthesiologist.

The real or actual cause(s) of the destabilization of the patients reported is unknown. What is known is that there were 1606 reported instances in a total report of 573,785 cardiopulmonary bypass procedures. The patient outcome included 21 patients who were permanently injured after operation and 133 patients who died. This was the largest number of deaths or permanent injuries out of all other reported accidents or complications. This category accounted for 29% of the reported patient deaths and was twice as great as the next largest category. In 62% of these cases the patient was placed back on cardiopulmonary bypass under emergency conditions.

The "protamine reaction" question aside, it is apparent that the immediate postbypass period is hazardous for the open-heart patient. It is also apparent that the perfusionist would be well advised not to be in any great hurry to disassemble the cardiopulmonary bypass circuit or to leave the operating room.

Reference has been made in this chapter, and other chapters of the book, to protocols. Protocols are important but, as with checklists, (see Chapter 4:CHECKLISTS), should be used in the proper perspective. Certainly, parts of a protocol are "written in granite" and should be. Parts such as drug administration by the perfusionist, communication with the surgeon, blood product and fluid administration by the perfusionist are not subject to debate during bypass.

General Erwin Rommel stated: "No plan survives contact with the enemy. If a plan gets you into battle, that is enough, after that fight by ear and eye and tactical sense like a duellist." Protocols are similar to plans. They provide a framework and cover some of the things that might occur during bypass. **Protocols can not detail every contingency or emergency that might arise during perfusion.** Perfusionists must use their eyes and ears and particularly their brains to logically solve perfusion problems. The perfusionist must rely on experience and deductive reasoning to extricate the patient and themselves from a perfusion crisis. Dependence solely on protocol may well create a perfusion failure. Protocols are devised from experience and experience includes the mistakes, accidents, and failures, but not all of them that are possible. It may well be that today's educational system provides too much emphasis on protocol and not enough stress on experience, deductive reasoning, logic, and self-reliance.

REFERENCES

1. Cervera AL, Moss G: Dilutional re-expansion with crystalloid after massive hemorrhage: Saline versus balanced electrolyte solution for maintenance of normal blood volume and arterial pH. J Trauma 15:498, 1975.
2. Metz S, Hacker J: Effect of dextrose-crystalloid priming solution on fluid requirements and urine output during cardiopulmonary bypass. T Heart Inst J 13:341, 1986.
3. Wukasch DC, Malloy KP, Rubio PA, Reed CC, Sandiford FM, Reul GJ, Milam JD, Cooley DA: Fat embolization resulting from median sternotomy. Texas Med 71:35, 1975.
4. Reed CC, Miller D, Stafford TB, McInnis RJ: Microemboli emmission of extracorporeal oxygenators. Les cahiers du CECEC 22:35, 1984.
5. Baudet EM, Leonelli V, Berty A, Laborde MN, Roques XF: Method for right atrial filling at the end of extracorporeal circulation. Perfusion 2: 223. 1987.
6. DeWall R: What constitutes adequate perfusion? J Cardiovasc Surg 16:458,1975.

..LAWSUITS AND ...CASENOTES

... The patient's femoral artery was cannulated for arterial return during cardiopulmonary bypass for aortocoronary bypass graft surgery. When bypass began the perfusion pressure fell to 15 mmHg and the surgeons observed the aorta spontaneously and abruptly widen from the diaphragm to the left ventricle. The perfusionist was not monitoring arterial line pressure but the arterial line began "thumping" slightly at the same time the aorta was observed to widen. The surgeons attempted to repair the dissected aorta, but the patient died from uncontrollable bleeding. Autopsy revealed that the dissection extended into the coronary arteries.

.. During mitral valve replacement the surgeon inserted the vent into the left atrium via the left superior pulmonary vein. Blood initially began to travel down the vent tubing toward the heart-lung machine, but then reversed direction and blew a large amount of air into the heart. The cross-clamp had not been applied at the time. The patient suffered severe neurological damage. Suit was filed against the perfusionist, the surgeon, and the hospital. The case was settled out of court for an amount in excess of $1,250,000.

... Bypass had been terminated and the patient was stable but slightly hypotensive. The perfusionist was instructed to infuse blood through the aortic cannula. The perfusionist failed to adequately monitor the arterial blood level and infused air into the patient's aorta. The patient was pronounced dead the following day.

... The perfusionist was slowly transfusing the contents of the oxygenator into the patient through the aortic cannula. The perfusionist leaned across the heart-lung machine to completely drain the venous line into the oxygenator and to re-clamp the venous line nearer the device. The perfusionist's knee moved the rheostat control knob unknowingly which increased the arterial pumphead RPM. The oxygenator emptied and air was transfused into the patient's aorta. The pump was reversed in an attempt to remove the air. The patient made an uneventful postoperative recovery.

... Towards the end of the operative procedure and while on partial cardiopulmonary bypass the anesthesiologist inadvertently gave protamine. The oxygenator contents of the oxygenator solidified and the patient was pronounced dead on the operating table.

... At the termination of bypass the contents of the oxygenator were transferred to IV bags and given to the anesthesiologist. During transfusion of this blood through a CVP line and using a pressure infusion cuff, a large amount of air was transfused into the patient from the half-full IV bag. The patient survived uninjured.

... During cardiopulmonary bypass the perfusionist also was required to operate the IABP. When the low level alarm sounded the perfusionist went to the balloon pump thinking it was that audible alarm which sounded very similar to the oxygenator low level alarm. Air was pumped into the patient who expired. The perfusionist was terminated from the job.

... One team reports two cases of arterial air emboli due to inattention to arterial reservoir level and two cases of arterial air emboli from unnoticed rotation of the arterial pumphead. No patient injuries resulted due to the open purge line on the arterial filter which vented the gas out of the arterial line.

... During an evening emergency redo-mitral valve replacement for the third time the perfusionist was rushed setting up the heart-lung machine. When the vent was threaded through the pumphead the perfusionist smashed a finger in the roller-head. The tubing slipped out of the raceway. The perfusionist reinserted the tubing and some few minutes later bypass was initiated. The surgeon inserted a right superior pulmonary vein vent and directed that the pump be turned on. He immediately complained that the vent was not working and the perfusionist increased the pump speed. The vent still failed to function properly and the perfusionist stopped the vent pump. At that point the surgeon asked if the vent line was properly threaded through the pumphead. The perfusionist checked and found the vent tubing inserted backwards through the pumphead. The surgeon had not applied the aortic cross-clamp prior to insertion of the vent and the patient received massive air emboli. The operative procedure was completed. The patient expired that evening.

.. During aortocoronary bypass graft surgery the perfusionist allowed the arterial reservoir level to fall and air was pumped into the patient. No low level alarms, bubble detector, or arterial line filter were used. At trial the perfusionist testified that the particular oxygenator he was using (a bubble oxygenator) could be operated with a level of 200 ml or even less because the design of the device prevented air from being vortexed under any circumstances. The jury found the perfusionist guilty of malpractice and the surgeon not negligent but liable for the actions of the perfusionist. The award was $650,000 to the plaintiff.

.. The perfusionist emptied the arterial reservoir during cardiopulmonary bypass for aortocoronary bypass graft surgery. The patient expired. Suit was filed against the hospital, surgeon, and perfusionist. At deposition it was determined that no safety devices were in use and that no arterial line filter was being used. It was also determined that two weeks earlier the same thing had occurred with the same perfusionist with the same results, the patient expired. The jury found for the plaintiff and awarded $600,000. The jury determined that the perfusionist was guilty of malpractice and that the surgeon was not negligent but was liable for the actions of the perfusionist.

.. During cardiopulmonary bypass for repair of a congenital defect in an adult patient the perfusionist emptied the oxygenator two and possibly three times during the case, pumping air into the patient on each occasion. There were no safety alarms being used and the arterial filter in the circuit had a stopcock on the purge port which was operated in the closed position. The jury awarded the plaintiff $375,000.

.. During cardiopulmonary bypass air was pumped into the patient through the arterial line. No safety alarms were being used nor was an arterial filter in the bypass circuit. The case settled out of court for an amount in excess of $850,000.

.. During aortocoronary bypass graft surgery the patient suffered moderate to severe brain damage. Ten years later he filed suit against the surgeon, the perfusionists, and the hospital. The hospital no longer existed, having been taken over by another hospital. The perfusionists could not be located. The records were minimal at best. The perfusion record and the anesthesia record indicated a bypass pressure at the start of bypass of approximately 35-43 mmHg for a period of less than 10 minutes, which plaintiff claimed was the cause of the brain damage. The patient had no history or evidence of carotid disease or cerebrovascular disease prior to surgery. The primary surgeon had relocated to the other side of the United States and by deposition the assistant surgeon was a self-proclaimed expert on perfusion who either knew very little about cardiopulmonary bypass or was unable to express his knowledge. Faced with these circumstances, and totally unable to locate even one of the perfusionists involved, the defense chose to settle the case for an amount in excess of $450,000 after a motion for dismissal under the statute of limitations had been denied.

Chapter 14:

PEDIATRIC CONSIDERATIONS

Chapter 14: PEDIATRIC CONSIDERATIONS

Pediatric perfusion is similar to adult perfusion only in principle. Unfortunately, most current devices for pediatric perfusion are scaled down versions of adult equipment, and some blood usually is required for priming the pediatric bypass circuit. Additionally, the surgical procedures during pediatric perfusion generally are more complex, and the bypass times required on cardiopulmonary bypass tend to be longer. Adjunctive techniques such as hypothermia, or deep hypothermia and circulatory arrest may also be utilized.

CHOICE OF OXYGENATOR

The authors are aware of no overwhelming advantages to either bubble or membrane type oxygenators when used for pediatric perfusion. There may be a tendency to think that because a membrane oxygenator is "theoretically superior" to a bubble oxygenator, then it is even more "theoretically superior" for the sick pediatric patient. This simply is not the case probably due to other factors inherent with conventional cardiopulmonary bypass and blood/foreign surface interactions.

Since the cardiac chambers are opened during pediatric perfusion, no closed system membrane oxygenator really exists. Besides, the vents and suckers aspirate large volumes of room air along with recovered blood. The pediatric patient's recovery after bypass is more dependant on the surgical repair than what type of oxygenator was used. The authors also believe that blood/foreign surface effects with current bypass devices are still poorly understood. Recent data indicate that pediatric patients may be more susceptible to the phenomenon of complement activation during cardiopulmonary bypass. Therefore, it is advisable to carefully consider the change to or addition of any new devices for pediatric perfusion (such as, a different membrane oxygenator or the addition of an ultrafiltration device) when conventional devices such as the bubble oxygenator have the benefit of long and successful clinical experience behind them. Additions and/or changes should be based on need, changing requirements, or failure or dissatisfaction with currently used devices. A glib salesman or attractive literature is no basis for change. The fact that a membrane oxygenator is requisite for prolonged ECMO applications does not necessarily mean it is superior for short duration bypass procedures in the infant patient (see Chapter 23: ECMO CIRCUITS AND TECHNIQUES).

CALCULATION OF PATIENT/PUMP HEMATOCRIT

A primary concern during pediatric perfusion is the ratio of required cardiopulmonary bypass circuit volume to patient blood volume. In adults the ratio is typically 1:3 (e.g., 2000 ml prime and 6000 ml estimated blood volume in the 75 kg patient). In children and infants the ratio often is 1:1 or less. In very small infants the pump priming volume may exceed the patient's blood volume by as much as 2:1 (e.g., 600 ml prime requirement and 300 ml blood volume in the 3.75 kg infant).

Several formulae have been used to calculate estimated blood volume (EBV) of pediatric patients. It must be recognized that these are only estimates and can vary by up to 10% of the patient's actual blood volume. The type of cardiac disease, prebypass fluid administration, or preoperative medications also significantly can affect the patient's blood volume.

One formula uses the factor 80 ml/kg to estimate blood volume regardless of patient size. Multiplying this value by the hematocrit gives the red cell volume (RCV) of the patient. Dividing the RCV by the sum of the EBV, required pump prime volume and estimated initial dose of cardioplegia gives a reasonable prediction of the initial mixed patient/pump hematocrit after initial infusion of cardioplegic solution. One important variable that is difficult to predict is the volume of IV fluid administered by the anesthesiologist prior to bypass. It is also important that the hematocrit used for making RCV calculations is a recent value. The effects of cardiac catheterization, diuresis, fluids (IV or PO), and length of NPO all can radically alter the pediatric patient's hematocrit at the time of bypass.

If the result of the calculation of the combined hematocrit is below protocol, or 22 to 25%, then packed cells or whole blood should be added to the bypass circuit prime. The hematocrit is approximately 75% for packed cells; for whole blood it is approximately 35%. Enough bank blood must be added to achieve the desired hematocrit.

For example, an 8 kg patient with a 46% hematocrit will be placed on cardiopulmonary bypass using a bypass circuit which has a total priming volume of 550 ml. The following calculations are made:

patient weight × factor	= EBV	8 × 80 = 640
EBV × patient hematocrit	= RCV	640 × .46(46%) = 294.4
EBV + bypass requirement + cardioplegia	= volume	640 + 550 + 150 = 1340
RCV ÷ volume = combined Hct		294.4 ÷ 1340 = .22 or 22%

If the same patient in the same circumstances had a hematocrit of 32% the calculations would be:

$$640 \times .32 = 204.8$$
$$204.8 \div 1340 = .15 \text{ or } 15\%$$

The mixed patient/pump hematocrit of 15% is too low. Therefore whole blood or packed cells are required in the prime. Adding packed cells, the calculations are as follows:

adding 50 ml	37.5 + 204.8 = 242.3 RCV
	pt/pump Hct = .18 or 18%
adding 50 ml	37.5 + 242.3 = 279.8 RCV
	pt/p Hct = .21 or 21%
adding 50 ml	37.5 + 279.7 = 317.3 RCV
	pt/p Hct = .24 or 24%

The mixed patient/pump hematocrit is acceptable and the cardiopulmonary bypass circuit is primed using 150 ml of packed cells. If whole blood was used instead, it would take 250 ml of whole blood to achieve a combined hematocrit of .22 or 22%.

Another method used to calculate the volume of blood to be added to the bypass circuit varies the RCV to be added based on the desired hematocrit. Such volumes of added blood, whether packed cells or whole, are variable. The authors believe it is simpler to use consistent numbers in 50 ml or 100 ml increments to arrive at or slightly above the desired hematocrit. In this way, reconstitution of blood or other prime additives are consistent and less prone to error.

Either technique may be used and the perfusionist can make appropriate adjustments in the formulae depending on the priming requirements of a particular circuit and the desired combined hematocrit.

Polycythemic patients whose calculated combined hematocrit is higher than desired should have extra crystalloid solution added to the prime, particularly if hypothermia is anticipated. Hematocrits greater than 30% on bypass can decrease tissue perfusion at lower temperatures due to red cell sludging and aggregation. A proposed rule of thumb states that the hematocrit on bypass should equal the degree Celsius of hypothermia employed, e.g., 20% at 20° C. This is for the pediatric patient.

RECONSTITUTION OF BLOOD

All bank blood added to the bypass circuit at any time should be reconstituted to compensate for changes that occur during storage. Packed cells are used in most pediatric patients. A method of reconstitution is:

300 units of heparin
3 mEq of sodium bicarbonate
60 mg of calcium chloride

These drugs, in these dosages, are added for *each* 50 ml of blood. The drugs should be added to the bypass circuit through the venous line to ensure adequate mixing and distribution. Calcium chloride is always added last.

If whole blood greater than 72 hours old is used, some teams increase the heparin dosage to 600 units of heparin per 50 ml of blood and the other drugs and dosages remain the same.

If fresh whole blood is used for infants less than six months of age, a method of reconstitution is for every 50 ml of blood is:

600 units heparin
1 mEq sodium bicarbonate
60 mg of calcium chloride

It is important when adding blood to the bypass circuit that calcium chloride be given last after adding heparin and that calcium chloride never be allowed to pool in the circuit. Calcium ions are an important component in the coagulation cascade, and cases have been reported of massive clots forming in the bypass circuit when the drug was added to bank blood that was not heparinized.

CANNULATION

Selection of properly sized cannulae is important in pediatric perfusion. Fortunately today there is a wide range of cannulae designed for the pediatric patient.

Some teams choose arterial cannulae based on a pressure drop of less than 100 mmHg. More practically, the surgeon chooses the largest cannula that may reasonably be inserted. Pressure drops for aortic cannulae are shown in Table 14.1.

Dual venous cannulae are most often used during congenital cardiac surgery to provide optimum operating conditions on the right side of the heart. Dual venous cannulae may be placed through the right atrium and into the SVC and IVC, or the cavae may be cannulated directly. If direct caval cannulation is used, right-angled, thin-walled cannulae may be used. Adequate venous return is easily obtained even in the smallest infants, and the direct caval cannulae usually do not obstruct the surgical field.

VENTING

Pediatric vents are used during bypass to aspirate blood or air from the heart. Operation of the vent pumphead is no different from adult cardiopulmonary bypass. It should be operated at the lowest possible speed to adequately remove blood without sucking in large volumes of room air. The volume aspirated through the vent may consist of a large portion of venous return to the oxygenator. It is important for the perfusionist to constantly be aware of the status of the vent. The surgeon should communicate removal of the vent since the absence of vent return can drastically alter the level in the arterial reservoir. The perfusionist should inform the surgeon if the vent becomes occluded.

Table 14.1 MAXIMUM RECOMMENDED BLOOD FLOW (L/MINUTE) PEDIATRIC ARTERIAL CANNULAE

Mfg.	Model	Size(OD)	Type	Flow
Argyle	591016	10 Fr	Str	0.65
DLP	75008	8 Fr	Str	0.7
DLP	75010	10 Fr	Str	1.0
Sarns	12308	14 Fr	Ang	1.5
Argyle	591032	14 Fr	Str	1.75
DLP	75014	14 Fr	Str	2.5
Sarns	12315	5.2 mm	Ang	3.5
Argyle	591057	18 Fr	Str	3.5

Note: 100 mmHg ΔP using tap water. Str = Straight; Ang = Angled.

CARDIOPLEGIA

Cardioplegia, when utilized, is administered in proportionately smaller doses. Two commonly used dosages are 450 ml/m^2 and 10 to 15 ml/kg. This can vary greatly from team to team. If the perfusionist administers cardioplegia from the pump it is often given through a large bore, hand-held needle inserted into the aorta by the surgeon. Some believe that it is important to know the pressure drop across the needle so as to keep the aortic root pressure about 60 mmHg. Such pressure is adequate for closing the aortic valve and perfusing the coronary arteries and decreases the risk of overpressurization of the heart.

HEMODYNAMICS

Hemodynamics during pediatric perfusion differ from those of adult perfusion. Lower perfusion pressures are produced during bypass and seem to be well tolerated by the pediatric patient. This is probably due to the hemodilution effect and lower peripheral resistance than is usually seen in the adult. It is not unusual to see the perfusion pressure fall to 25 to 30 mmHg in the first few minutes of bypass even at perfusion rates of 80 to 100 ml/kg or 2.4 to 2.6 L/min/m.^{2}

Because of smaller blood volumes in the patient and bypass circuit, dramatic changes in the patient's hemodynamics occur in response to small changes in oxygenator reservoir levels. A translocation of only 25 to 50 ml in either direction can make the difference between a heart that is ejecting and one that is not. The perfusionist must be particularly aware of these small changes in reservoir volumes. Venous drainage in the pediatric patient is important since sustained elevated venous pressures can cause cerebral or hepatic damage. The anesthesiologist can best assist with assessment of venous drainage. The surgeon should always be informed of poor venous return. If no mechanical cause can be found, the problem may be addressed by adding small volumes of fluid, or reducing blood flow. If the patient is cooled, a small reduction in blood flow should present no problem.

BLOOD GASES

Blood gases are regulated the same as they are during adult perfusion. One difference is that pediatric oxygenators tend to be overly efficient because of the size of the patient. It is sometimes more difficult to regulate blood gases during infant perfusion, and it is not unusual to see the pO_2 in the higher 300 to 400 mmHg ranges and the pCO_2s in the lower range of 25 to 30 mmHg. The use of inline blood gas monitors may provide better control over the blood gases in the pediatric patient and may even justify their existence and expense in this setting.

HYPOTHERMIA AND CIRCULATORY ARREST

This topic is discussed in detail in Chapter 16. During pediatric perfusion the same principles apply, and the primary consideration is that the pediatric patient's temperature response is more rapid than the adult in both cooling and rewarming. The gradient between the patient temperature and the arterial blood must be no greater than 8°C when cooling or rewarming. When rewarming, the temperature gradient is measured between the venous blood and the heat exchanger control unit.

Temperature measurements differ in the pediatric patient because often the naso-pharyngeal, esophageal, or bladder probes are not placed. Tympanic membrane tempera-ture measurements are the most practical.

..LAWSUITS AND ...CASENOTES

... During pediatric cardiopulmonary bypass the perfusion team used heat lamps positioned to shine directly on the arterial line between the oxygenator and the patient. During operation gas bubbles were noted in the arterial line. The pump was stopped and the bubbles cleared. The bubbles recurred and it was determined that the hot lights were causing gas bubbles to come out of solution due to the temperature gradient. There was no injury to the patient.

... During circulatory arrest tiny gas bubbles were seen to accumulate in the top of the arterial tubing. The patient died at surgery of other complications. It was found that the oxygenator, a scaled down version of the adult model, had a design defect built in during size reduction. That model oxygenator was discontinued although the manufacturer did not recall the product and denied the defect existed.

... A new model infant bubble oxgenator was used on a 5.5 kg infant with an A-V canal. The patient was cooled to 24° C, which took 30 minutes. After surgical correction of the defect the perfusionist began rewarming. It took nearly 60 minutes for the patient's temperature, measured tympanically, to reach 35° C. The patient bled excessively postoperatively and had significant hematuria. The patient expired. It was discovered that the internal part which distributed venous blood over the heat exchanger coil was defective and permitted blood to pass directly through the defoamer bypassing the heat exchanger.

Chapter15:

PERFUSION ACID-BASE BALANCE

Chapter 15: PERFUSION ACID-BASE BALANCE

The basic purpose of perfusion, physiologically, whether in the intact organism or by an artificial heart-lung machine, is to provide all perfused tissues with oxygen (needed for cell metabolism) and to remove carbon dioxide (produced by cell metabolism). The development of metabolic acidosis in patients on cardiopulmonary bypass was routinely observed during early clinical experience. There were several reasons for this phenomenon which undoubtedly was due in part to use of devices (oxygenators and pumps) that were less efficient than those currently available. Contributing factors were the use of whole blood primes and less than optimum anesthetic management. A fundamental problem, too, was in obtaining meaningful blood gas analysis during cardiopulmonary bypass which was often delayed, and once received, poorly understood. It was not unusual to receive results of samples drawn during bypass after the patient was in ICU, or even 24 hours later. Further obscuring the situation, the ideal flow rates were debated then, just as they are debated now. The success of Lillehei using cross-circulation and the "azygos flow principle"[1] which advocated very low flow rates led many teams to adopt the technique of low flow perfusion.

By the early 1960s, however, it became recognized that the development of metabolic acidosis during bypass was due to poor tissue perfusion due to these low flow rates, and that the lower the flow during perfusion the more marked was the fall in the buffer base.[2]

Fortunately, the days of progressive metabolic acidosis and administering multiple boluses of sodium bicarbonate almost empirically on a time schedule are but a memory. Hemodilution perfusion, better anesthetic management, and refined oxygenators and pumps have virtually eliminated this problem.

What has not been resolved, however, is a clear understanding of how to achieve or even measure optimum acid-base balance during cardiopulmonary bypass. While the trend towards the "alpha stat" method of blood gas control appears to be growing in popularity, it is not nearly practiced universally. The Survey revealed that approximately two-thirds of the respondents routinely temperature corrected blood gas results (pH-stat methodology) while one-third did not (alpha-stat methodology).

If it were simply a difference between correcting or not correcting blood gas values, the technique of gas management would be analogous to driving a car on the right-hand side of the road versus the left-hand side: doing it either way gets you to your destination, but the perspective is slightly different. Both techniques ideally strive for an arterial pH of 7.40 and a pCO_2 of 40 mmHg. However, not temperature correcting the blood gas will result in elevated pCO_2 and pO_2 values for those used to temperature correcting.

The fundamental difference between the pH-stat and alpha-stat approach only becomes apparent during hypothermia. When blood is cooled the pCO_2 naturally decreases and the pH naturally increases. The rationale for the pH-stat technique in which carbon dioxide is added to the oxygenator to counteract the fall in pH is two-fold: 1) it prevents cerebral vasoconstriction and presumably maintains cerebral perfusion, and 2) it counteracts the tendency of the oxyhemoglobin dissociation curve to shift left which decreases O_2 availability. Using the pH-stat technique with temperature corrected blood gases, CO_2 is added to the oxygenator gas to keep the pH at 7.40, regardless of temperature. Using the alpha-stat technique with uncorrected blood gases (measured at 37° C), CO_2 is not added unless the pCO_2 falls excessively (e.g., <25 mmHg), although Swan has recently advocated an "exaggerated" alpha-stat technique in which venous blood gases should be highly alkaline (pH 7.8 to 7.9, pCO_2 15 to 20 mmHg).[3] The authors are aware of no clinical studies that confirm the benefits of this technique and, in fact, even with current highly efficient oxygenators, achieving this level of alkalinity during bypass is difficult.

The key issue is the CO_2 content of blood which ideally should remain constant regardless of body temperature.[4] If the total blood CO_2 content remains constant the bicarbonate buffer system will keep the pH in the proper range. Because the "proper" range of pH is referenced to neutrality, the pH will naturally rise with decreasing temperature. Adding CO_2 and "correcting" the blood gas to achieve a pH of 7.4 and pCO_2 of 40 mmHg will, in fact, be artificially increasing the total blood CO_2 content and cause CO_2 retention and metabolic acidosis which must be compensated for by increasing the perfusion flow rate. Using the alpha-stat technique, the pCO_2 will fall as the temperature is decreased.

The fear of decreased cerebral blood flow has not been borne out by using this technique, and cerebral autoregulation may be better maintained without the addition of CO_2.[5-7] Adding CO_2 to the oxygenator, in fact, has been shown to have a deleterious effect on myocardial preservation,[3] which, of course, has little importance during cardioplegic arrest.

Practically, the alpha-stat technique is accomplished more easily than the pH-stat technique by not adding any CO_2 to the oxygenator. The pCO_2 should be kept at 30 to 40 mmHg regardless of temperature using alpha-stat as derived from an "uncorrected" blood gas. Upon rewarming, the pH will come down to 7.4 without the addition of sodium bicarbonate, (see Figure 15.1.) If the pH-stat technique is followed, with CO_2 added during hypothermia to maintain the pH at 7.4, the oxygenator must be "hyperventilated" during rewarming to remove the excess CO_2 and blood flow rates must be increased to reverse the metabolic acidosis. Using the car analogy again, besides the difference in perspective

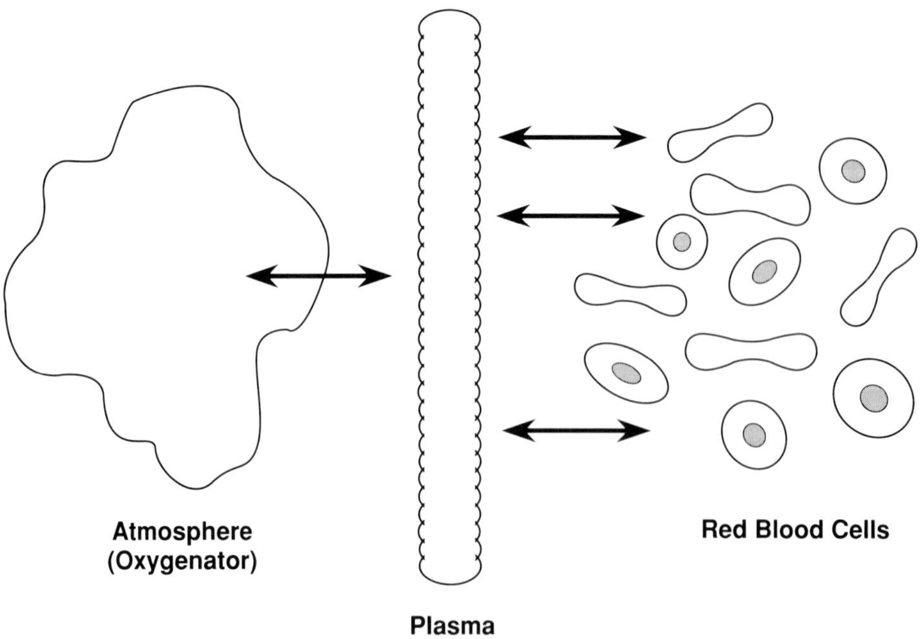

Figure 15.1 Gas equilibrium between red blood cells, plasma, and atmosphere inside the oxygenator.

regarding blood gas results, the pH-stat car is a standard shift while the alpha-stat car has an automatic transmission, thus the driver (perfusionist) must work harder using pH-stat management.

If metabolic acidosis develops during cardiopulmonary bypass, perfusion is inadequate, meaning the ratio of oxygen needed by the tissue to the amount supplied to the tissue is not in balance. Administering sodium bicarbonate will not correct this fundamental inadequacy, but it will increase the pH. This is akin to treating the symptoms and not the disease and only will result in changing the blood gas numbers, but little else. Metabolic acidosis can cause peripheral vasoconstriction and elevated perfusion pressures which may lead to a false sense that perfusion is satisfactory. Sodium bicarbonate will sometimes transiently lower the perfusion pressure and is no cause for alarm. A guideline for the amount of $NaHCO_3$ to add for a given base deficit is to multiply the patient's weight in kg by the deficit and 0.3. The result will indicate how many mEq of $NaHCO_3$ to add to raise the pH to 7.40. In practice this formula should be used cautiously as hypothermia slows HCO_3 transport across cell membranes and metabolic alkalosis can result.

A more useful guide regarding perfusion acid-base balance is measuring the mixed venous pO_2 which should be greater than 25 mmHg (ideally 30 to 40 mmHg) *at all times* in the adequately perfused patient. Using the alpha-stat method, the venous pO_2, in fact, often becomes markedly elevated during hypothermia.

Analysis of sample blood for blood gas determinations actually measures the amount of each separate gas which exist as gas dissolved in the plasma of the blood. It does not measure the amount of gas, or the partial pressure of the various gases, contained in the whole blood itself or contained in or on the red blood cells. A gas equilibrium exists between the red blood cells and the plasma. The equilibrium is driven towards the red blood cell as long as excess gas is dissolved in the plasma (see Figure 15.1).

Hemoglobin has a higher affinity for oxygen than it does for carbon dioxide. Thus, as long as oxygen is dissolved in the plasma, carbon dioxide will be given up by the hemoglobin molecule and oxygen will affix itself to the hemoglobin. Carbon dioxide which then exists as dissolved gas must equilibrate with the atmosphere inside the oxygenator.

Until the mid-1960s the direct measurement of pO_2 and pCO_2 was not possible. Measurement of O_2 content had to be performed and the percent saturation calculated. When direct measurement of oxygen and carbon dioxide tensions became available, the entire open-heart field changed over to this measurement technique because it was more accurate and more rapid. When the first commercially available membrane oxygenators reached the marketplace they performed so poorly that they achieved no sales success. In spite of all the tricks possible to increase oxygenating efficiency, such as preheating the oxygen, pressurizing the membrane and squeezing the blood path, and partially recirculating through the oxygenator a second time, the early membranes could not produce pO_2s equal to that of the bubble oxygenators. To overcome this defect, the membrane manufacturers re-introduced the concept of oxygen saturation, a distinct retrograde step in perfusion. Perfusionists missed the point entirely. A saturation of 97% is about equal to a pO_2 of 97 mmHg, while a saturation of 99% is equal to a pO_2 of 180 mmHg. In other words, the early membranes could not produce a pO_2 of 100 mmHg. Percent saturation has no place in perfusion today. To use arterial pO_2 and then venous saturation is ludicrous.

Measuring venous O_2 saturation is a poor way to determine flow rates because the O_2 saturation reflects oxygen bound to hemoglobin. Measuring pO_2s is much more accurate.

Another often overlooked factor in acid-base balance is the level of anesthesia. The patient who is asleep but shivering due to bypass hypothermia will have an increased O_2 demand and consumption. This increased O_2 consumption must be met with adequate perfusion flows if metabolic acidosis is to be avoided. Observing the blood to darken without any change in flow rate or temperature is a clue that the patient may be shivering or becoming "light." A blood gas sample will confirm if the observation is valid.

Bank blood, albumin or non-pH adjusted crystalloids added to the bypass circuit, either in the prime or during bypass, should be buffered with $NaHCO_3$. For blood 3 mEq/50 ml and for albumin 5 mEq/50 ml will reduce the acid load to the patient. For crystalloids, 50 mEq/liter is sufficient. Alternatively, decreasing the arterial pCO_2 will raise the pH and partially compensate for the acid load that accompanies such fluid administration.

In clinical practice, regulation of blood gases during bypass has been the subject of controversy and confusion to the present,[8,9] and the belief that the maintenance of "physiological levels" of arterial pCO_2 and pO_2 (i.e., about 40 mmHg and 80 to 90 mmHg, respectively) ought to be the goal, is not supported by clinical experiences. However, this does not mean that the gas flow meter can be operated with abandon so long as the arterial blood is bright red during perfusion. Recent information concerning gaseous microemboli, particularly when bubble oxygenators are used, indicate that sagacious perfusion practice would strive for a pO_2 less than 200 mmHg and above 100 mmHg. The pCO_2 should be maintained between 35 and 45 mmHg using the alpha-stat method of blood gas control.

In summary, assessment of venous pO_2, arterial pCO_2 and pO_2, hemoglobin, and perfusion rate are necessary for evaluation of perfusion adequacy. Adequate flow, adequate gas exchange, and an adequate hematocrit are necessary for adequate perfusion.

REFERENCES

1. Andreasen AT, Watson F: Experimental cardiovascular surgery: "The azygos factor." Br J Surg 39:548, 1952.
2. Galletti PM, Brecher GA: Metabolic aspects of total heart-lung bypass. Ch 14 in *Heart-Lung Bypass, Principles and Techniques of Extracorporeal Circulation*. New York: Grune & Stratton, 1962.
3. Swan H: The importance of acid-base management for cardiac and cerebral preservation during open-heart operations. Surg Gynecol Obstet 158:391, 1984.
4. Ream AK, Reitz BA, Silverberg G: Temperature corrections of pCO_2 and pH in estimating acid-base status:An example of the emperor's new clothes? Anesthesiol 56:41, 1982.
5. Norwood WI, Norwood CR, Castaneda AR: Cerebral anoxia: Effect of deep hypothermia and pH. Surg 86:203, 1979.
6. Fox LS, Blackstone EH, Kirklin JW, Stewart RW, Samuelson PN: Relationship of whole body oxygen consumption to perfusion flow rate during hypothermic cardiopulmonary bypass. J Thorac Cardovasc Surg 83:239, 1982.
7. Williams JJ, Marshall BE: Editorial: A fresh look at an old question. Anesthesiol 56:1, 1982.
8. Kurusz M, Butler BD: Oxygenator performance influence on clinical decisions. Perfusion 1:213, 1986.
9. Pearson DT, Holden MP, Poslad SJ, Murray A, Waterhouse PS: Reply. Perfusion 1:214, 1986.
10. Penido JRF, Swan HJC, Kirklin JW:Oxygen content of blood arterialized in bubble-type plastic sheet oxygenators (an experimental study). Proceed Mayo Clin 32:389, 1957.
11. Effler DB, Kolff WJ, Groves LK: Complications peculiar to open-heart surgery. Surg 45:149, 1959.

..LAWSUITS AND ...CASENOTES

... During cardiopulmonary bypass the blood gas samples showed profound hypoxia. Efforts to correct the problem were unsuccessful until the perfusionist, who had not set up the cardiopulmonary bypass circuit, removed the clamp from the gas line.

Chapter16:

HYPOTHERMIA AND CIRCULATORY ARREST

Chapter 16: HYPOTHERMIA AND CIRCULATORY ARREST

Systemic hypothermia is nearly universally used in some form and to some degree in conjunction with cardiopulmonary bypass. Hypothermia offers several advantages to the patient during cardiac surgery. By decreasing oxygen demand it permits the tolerance of periods of reduced flow and is an additional measure of safety for the patient in the event total circulatory arrest is required. The predominant physiological advantage of hypothermia, however, is that oxygen requirements of the patient are decreased which allows toleration of lower blood flows during bypass.

While hypothermia has the benefit of vast clinical experience dating in cardiac surgery from the 1950s, an understanding of the precise physiologic mechanisms that are involved is lacking. Such an understanding appears to be of less interest to the perfusionist who is more concerned with the technical aspects for safely inducing and reversing hypothermia during cardiopulmonary bypass.

Levels of hypothermia are based on surgical preference and generally depend on both the type and anticipated length of the operative procedure. Systemic hypothermia permits the surgeon wider flexibility in manipulating blood flows if blood at the operative site interferes with the operation. Hypothermia also has the added benefit of decreasing the gradient between the cold arrested heart and the body temperature during cardioplegia. Even with the aorta cross-clamped there is a tendency for the heart to rewarm due to collateral blood flow, bronchial blood flow, and the proximity of adjacent warmer organs and tissues which surround it. Systemic hypothermia can slow this process.

TEMPERATURE GRADIENTS

In the development of perfusion equipment, manufacturers have demonstrated the ability to build highly efficient disposable heat exchangers, most of which are integral to the oxygenator. The efficiency of these heat exchangers have greatly exceeded physiological or practical needs, and appear to have been developed for reasons other than safety, perhaps a demand for speed. These highly efficient heat exchangers must be used with great caution in order to avoid damage to blood, tissues, and organs of the body when inducing hypothermia or rewarming.

An appreciation of the importance of temperature gradients between the perfused tissue and the heat exchanger is a fundamental principle taught to perfusionists. Perfusion rewarming from hypothermia with bubble oxygenators, if the heat exchanger temperature is maximally warm can induce gas bubbles to come out of solution. Also, if the heat exchanger temperature is permitted to rise above 43 to 45° C, significant hemolysis can result and is manifested primarily by hemoglobinuria and secondarily by bleeding.

Additionally, and more ominously, **if the heat exchanger temperature exceeds the blood temperature by more than 10° C, gas bubbles can form in the perfusate as gas comes out of solution.**[1] More insidiously, deleterious effects may occur when patients are cooled with similarly excessive gradients.

The location in the bypass circuit of early, non-disposable heat exchangers was in the arterial line and after the oxygenator. This is an appropriate location when cooling, but not for rewarming the blood. Oxygenator manufacturers soon realized that one cause of the reported problems was this location, and the heat exchanger was designed into the bubble oxygenator oxygenating column before blood passed through the defoamer. The rationale was that any gas bubbles liberated during rewarming would be removed by passage through the defoamer. However, during induction of hypothermia, the cold blood is rewarmed by the patient's body. So, this makes it appear of little practical importance where the heat exchanger is located. What is important is how the heat exchanger is used.

The important technique consideration with perfusion hypothermia is that excessive gradients between the heat exchanger and perfusate or patient must be avoided. This means that when *cooling* the temperature of the perfusate should be regulated so as not to be lower than **7 to 10° C** below that of the patient. Exceeding this gradient when cooling can lead to red cell sludging, capillary bed shut down and shunting, and a tendency for gas to come out of solution as cold blood is warmed by the body. When *warming*, the same gradients, **7 to 10° C**, are observed by measuring venous blood temperature and heat exchanger water temperature.

Of course, surgical protocol or operative conditions may dictate that these reasonably outlined guidelines be exceeded and that, of course, is a medical decision. One reported technique consists of cooling maximally with the perfusate at 5° C upon initiation of cardiopulmonary bypass. In a series of 36 patients perfused in this manner the postoperative neurological complication rate was 17%.[2] If one chooses to ignore safe gradients they must be willing to accept such unreasonable risks. The risk exposure of the practitioner is only outweighed by the risk the patient is exposed to.

It is also important that the heat exchanger never be allowed to exceed 42° C as red cell damage will occur at 44° C. Maintaining this two degree safety margin provides protection if there are any errors in temperature probe accuracy or inattention on the part of the team and perfusionist. Some of the newer self-contained cooler/heater modules are limited in such a way as to make it impossible to exceed 42° C. All heat exchanger control units should be limited to 42° C maximum temperature. Not exceeding 42° C in the heat exchanger will rarely cause the perfusate temperature to exceed 39° C which is considered to be the upper safe limit. In smaller patients or pediatric patients, it is possible to exceed 39° C, so the perfusionist must carefully monitor perfusate temperature the entire time during rewarming.

During cooling, the perfusionist should begin reducing the cooling gradient when the patient is one or two degrees above the desired temperature to prevent the patient from drifting too low. During rewarming, which generally takes longer, the perfusionist may become preoccupied with other related activities. It is important that the patient not drift above the desired temperature and become over warmed. Increased attention to the heat control unit is required during this part of the bypass procedure.

Figure 16.1 illustrates graphically a typical safe "staged" cooling and rewarming technique.

BLOOD GASES

Blood gases during hypothermia should be maintained within ranges which are no different from those at normothermia. The physiological response of the patient to hypothermia is to have decreased pCO_2s due to less CO_2 production and elevated pO_2s due to decreased O_2 consumption. Appropriate adjustments in the gas flow and composition of the gases delivered to the oxygenator can minimize these tendencies.

BLOOD FLOW

Arterial flow rate should be maintained at 40-60 ml/kg/min or 2.2 to 2.4 L/min/m,[2] which is approximately 75% of normal cardiac output during cooling and rewarming. Reducing flow when cooling may prevent organ systems from being adequately cooled.

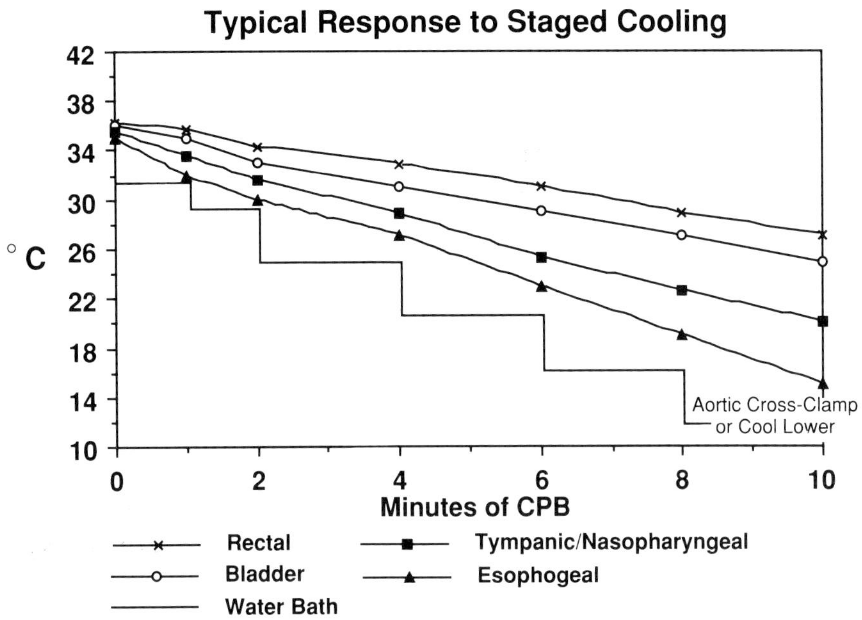

Note: Patient temperature is rarely 37 °C at initiation of CPB. Response of patient temperatures depends on flow rate, patient BSA, and target temperature. The temperature gradient never should exceed 7-10 °C.

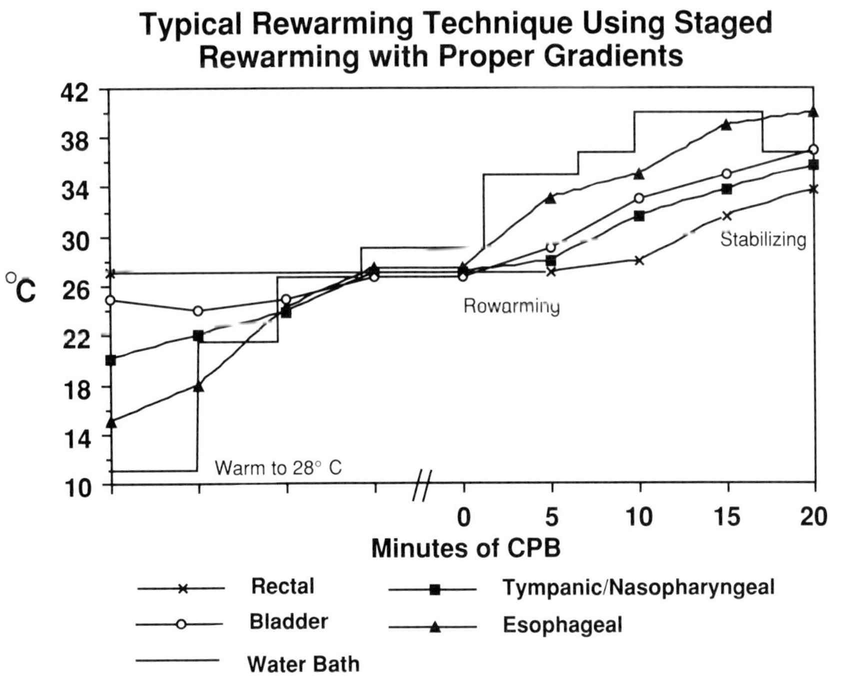

Note: Water bath temperature never exceeds 42 °C. Rewarm time varies with flow rate and patient BSA, and level of hypothermia. The temperature gradient never should exceed 7-10 °C.

Figure 16.1 Staged cooling and rewarming technique showing monitored temperatures.

Generally it takes 15 to 30 minutes at these flow rates to thoroughly cool the patient. This is governed by patient size and method of temperature monitoring.

When the patient is cold, oxygen consumption is reduced which may permit significant reductions in blood flow. Other schools of thought suggest that perfusion blood flows should remain unchanged, despite the lower temperature, and be governed only by venous return. Either technique has successful clinical outcomes and hundreds of thousands of patients have been safely perfused using both techniques.

Prematurely terminating bypass before the patient is adequately warmed can lead to temperature drifts downward in the postoperative period resulting in shivering and hypertension, both of which increase O_2 consumption and workload on the heart as it attempts to meet the metabolic demand.

PERFUSATE COMPOSITION

Hemodilution perfusion is a well accepted technique for many reasons and particularly nowadays with the added risk of transmission of AIDS from banked blood. Blood viscosity increases with hypothermia and thus hematocrits ranging into the high teens are acceptable when hypothermia to a patient temperature of 18 to 20° C is used. Perfusion techniques to avoid excessive hemodilution include prebypass calculations of mixed patient/perfusate hematocrit and routine hemoglobin or hematocrit measurements on bypass (see Chapter 14: PEDIATRIC CONSIDERATIONS). If blood is required, it is added during the rewarming period.

MONITORING

Accurate temperature monitoring during hypothermia is essential. The venous and arterial perfusate temperatures should be monitored, as well as the heat exchanger control unit. Patient temperatures that may be monitored include: esophageal, nasopharyngeal, tympanic, rectal, bladder, skin, and myocardium.

None of the listed sites will record the same temperature due to non-uniform rates of cooling and warming of the body. The esophageal temperature is most closely related to arterial blood temperature due to its proximity to the aorta. Nasopharyngeal and tympanic temperatures are considered to most nearly reflect brain temperature and are preferred whenever circulatory arrest or low-flow perfusion are used. The rectal temperature is the slowest to respond and the least reliable. A recent addition to temperature monitoring is the bladder probe incorporated in a urinary drainage catheter. The correlation to esophageal or nasopharyngeal is good, but it is subject to drift with urine output. Pulmonary artery temperature may be monitored with a Swan Ganz catheter and correlates to esophageal temperature. Skin probes have no demonstrated benefit during cardiopulmonary bypass.

Finally, myocardial temperature may be monitored to assess the effectiveness of cold cardioplegia infusion and as an indicator of when additional cold cardioplegia is needed to maintain the myocardium at the desired temperature. This monitoring method is more sensitive than observing electrical fibrillation on the ECG monitor.

CIRCULATORY ARREST

In a few cases cardiopulmonary bypass is suspended during operation. These procedures usually involve small infants in whom the venous cannulation or blood in the operative field interferes with the operation or adults in whom aortic arch surgery is performed. The technique occasionally is used on other procedures such as extensive vascular tumor resection or neurosurgery.

Surface cooling can be used as an adjunct in hypothermia on rare occasions. Surface cooling of the patient takes place after intubation and insertion of monitoring lines and IV lines, but prior to prepping the skin. The patient is cooled to 26 to 29° C and sometimes lower before surgery begins or cannulation occurs.

The usual noticeable effect is that the heart rate will slow. If the heart fibrillates unexpectedly the perfusionist must be ready to begin bypass immediately. In the absence of this situation, the patient is prepped and draped in the usual manner and the bypass lines are brought to the table. Cardiopulmonary bypass proceeds in the usual fashion and hypothermia continues on bypass until the desired systemic temperature is reached. When instructed by the surgeon the arterial pump is stopped and the arterial line is clamped. The venous line may be clamped or left unclamped to exsanguinate venous blood from the patient after the arterial perfusion pump is turned off.

In cardiopulmonary bypass there are few absolutes, and the "safe" period of circulatory arrest is no exception. The generally accepted period at a temperature of 18 to 20° C is 60 minutes and possibly is no greater than 45 minutes.[3] Circulatory arrest times are not a function of the perfusionist except to record the times and to inform the surgeon of elapsed time, if it is desired.

Prior to reestablishing cardiopulmonary bypass the aortic cannula should be inspected for air bubbles. Perfusion is reestablished with the heat exchanger control unit temperature near that of the patient. Rewarming is accomplished as previously described.

Some controversy exists as to whether the perfusate should be slowly recirculated during the period of circulatory arrest or simply permitted to stand and stagnate. The authors are unaware of any objective studies of this question. Logic would favor some recirculation to prevent a settling effect in the arterial reservoir of red cells with possible sludging or agglutination, particularly if an arterial filter is used. Certainly gas flow to the oxygenator should be reduced, but **never turned off.**

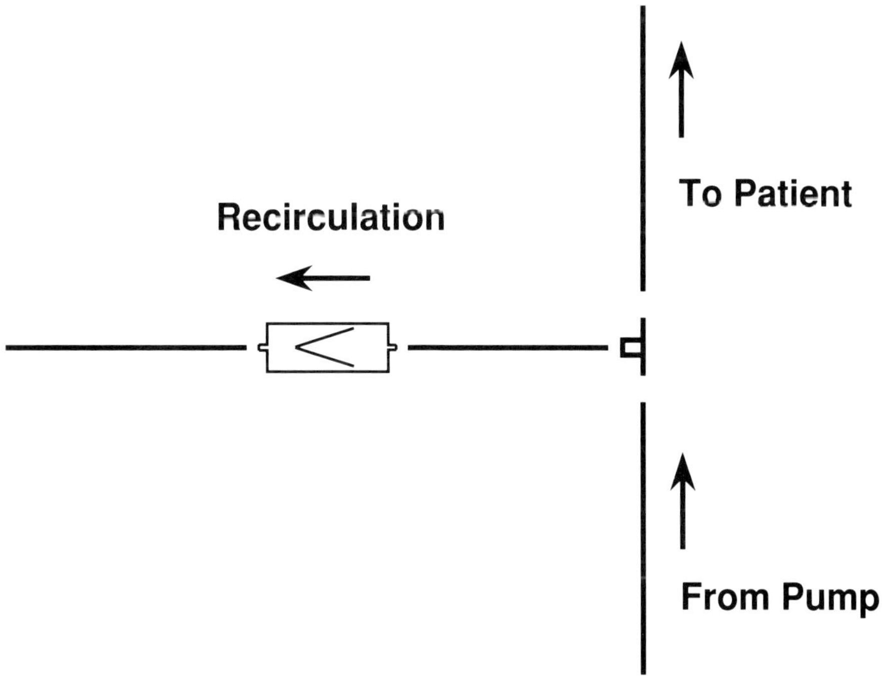

Figure 16.2 Recirculation line with one-way valve.

On infant set-ups one technique is to recirculate via a one-way valved line placed in a connector with a luer port and located distal to the arterial filter. The distal end of the purge line is returned to a low pressure site on the oxygenator (see Figure 16.2). Using this technique, one is assured that blood does not remain static in the arterial filter.

REFERENCES

1. Almond CH, Jones JC, Snyder HM, Grant SM, Meyer BW: Cooling gradients and brain damage with deep hypothermia. J Thorac Cardiovasc Surg 48:890, 1964.
2. Mahony L, Turley K, Ebert P, Heymann MA: Long-term results after arterial repair of transposition of the great arteries in early infancy. Am J Cardiol 50:637, 1982.
3. Kirklin JW, Barratt-Boyes B: Hypothermia, circulatory arrest and cardiopulmonary bypass. *Cardiac Surgery*, New York: John Wiley and Son, 1985.

..LAWSUITS AND ...CASENOTES

.. During repair of a transposition of great vessels in a pediatric patient, the patient was cooled with a torpedo heat exchanger to 23° C esophageally. Less than 15 minutes later the perfusionist was instructed by the surgeon to come off bypass. After surgical repair, bypass was resumed, the patient was rewarmed, and removed from bypass. Postoperatively the patient was discovered to have a significant neurological injury which necessitated 24 hour nursing care. Suit was filed by the parents against the surgeon, the hospital, and the manufacturer of the heart-lung machine. Jury found in favor of the plaintiff in excess of $1,000,000. The jury found the surgeon and the hospital negligent.

... During repair of an arch aneurysm, using deep hypothermia and circulatory arrest, neither the arterial nor venous lines were clamped during the arrest period. After the repair was completed, the patient was placed in the Trendelenburg position to evacuate air from the aorta. Unbeknownst to the surgeon, a large amount of air had entered the aorta during resection and traveled antegrade into the thoracic aorta. When bypass was restarted, air traveled retrograde into the cerebral vessels from the pressure and blood flow from the femoral artery cannula. The patient suffered severe neurological damage.

... During circulatory arrest the perfusate was not recirculated in the bypass circuit. The light on the heart-lung machine was in close proximity to the arterial line and apparently rewarmed the cold blood to the extent that multiple bubbles formed in the line from dissolved gas in the blood coming out of solution. The outcome is unknown.

Chapter 17:

PHARMACOLOGY OF BYPASS

Chapter 17: PHARMACOLOGY OF BYPASS

Just as in any major surgical procedure, pharmacology is an indispensable part of the patient management, and it is no different during cardiopulmonary bypass. It is also a fact that the decision to utilize drugs and/or to order their administration is limited to a licensed medical practitioner and not perfusionists, who generally only have rudimentary exposure to pharmacology during their training.

The Survey revealed, somewhat disturbingly, that approximately 20% of the perfusionists responding reportedly gave drugs of their own volition during cardiopulmonary bypass and without any physician's order or, more importantly, knowledge. **These authors are adamantly opposed to this practice.** Besides the question of legality, perfusionists may well think that the period of time the patient is on cardiopulmonary bypass is the most important period, but the pre and postbypass periods when the patient is anesthetized are perhaps even more important. Indeed the entire postoperative recovery period may be profoundly influenced by what drugs were given or not given or how they were given or not given in the operating room.

Human error in drug administration is a well-documented risk during anesthesia.[1,2] It is quite easy to predict that similar errors would be made by the busy perfusionist trying to manage blood flows, gas flows, blood gas analysis, and patient temperatures as is the common situation during cardiopulmonary bypass.

The influence of pharmacology on cardiopulmonary bypass techniques is limited. The balance of this chapter will briefly describe common drugs that are used during bypass and how they possibly affect cardiopulmonary bypass.

DRUGS WHICH AFFECT COAGULATION

The most important pharmacologic manipulation that permits conventional cardiopulmonary bypass, of course, is heparin anticoagulation. Dosages vary according to protocol, and it is well established that patient response may vary significantly[3,4] which has led to the near universal practice of monitoring the patient's coagulation status with either activated clotting times or heparin titration technology.[5] The authors believe that ACT monitoring is the preferable technique. The only obvious effect on bypass is if heparin anticoagulation is inadequate: in this situation clotting may occur in the bypass circuit with the risk of either plugging the bypass devices or causing embolization to the patient (see Chapter 12: MONITORING).

It should be noted that maintaining the ACT greater than 400 or 500 seconds *does not* assure one that the patient is adequately anticoagulated. Platelet aggregation still can occur in the cardiopulmonary bypass circuit with consumption of clotting factors (both cellular and acellular) if heparin levels are too low, and will prolong the ACT into the "safe" range.[6]

Until that time when some form of continuous and reliable inline assessment device or technique is devised to monitor heparin anticoagulation on a minute-by-minute basis, intermittent measurement of the ACT is a reasonable technique to reasonably assure the patient's blood will not clot while on cardiopulmonary bypass.

Heparin-induced thrombocytopenia is a phenomenon that has been described,[7,8] and it most often occurs in patients who have been receiving heparin for several days. Associated manifestations may include thromboembolic complications due to formation of platelet aggregates.[9] Perfusion techniques for these patients are no different than for those without the disorder.

"Heparin resistance" has been described in patients who are septic[10] or who are receiving heparin therapy prior to open-heart surgery.[11] Detection of this condition often is only by decreased ACT results with usual heparin dosages.

Patients who have taken drugs such as aspirin or dipyridamole (Persantine) preoperatively to decrease platelet adhesiveness will tend to bleed more during their surgery and particularly following bypass due to the added platelet trauma inherent with current cardiopulmonary bypass devices and techniques. However, a low platelet count or a prolonged bleeding time do not affect bypass techniques per se.

VASOCONSTRICTING DRUGS

Drugs given to counteract hypotension such as epinephrine (Adrenalin), norepinephrine (Levophed), ephedrine (Ephedrine Sulfate), dopamine (Intropin; Dopastat), phenylephrine (Neosynephrine) and others, will only affect bypass minimally and generally are manifested by increased reservoir volumes and higher perfusion pressures. If the effects are excessive (perfusion pressures > 100 mmHg) the perfusionist may temporarily decrease the flow to avoid prolonged hypertension. Significantly increasing the arterial reservoir level by translocating fluid from the patient will have the same effect, but this effect will be more gradual in occurrence.

VASODILATING DRUGS

Administration of vasodilators during bypass have the opposite effect of vasoconstrictors. The perfusion pressure will fall and more importantly, the oxygenator arterial reservoir level may fall to dangerously low levels as blood is translocated into the patient. Since these results can be abrupt and dramatic, the perfusionist should always be informed by the anesthesiologist if vasodilators are being administered. This policy may induce consternation in some, however, the separate teams must interact effectively (see Chapter 3: INTERFACE) since the actions of one may drastically influence **safe performance** of the other, and a human life may hang in the balance of non-communication. As with the previously listed drugs, vasodilators do not affect perfusion techniques per se, but may precipitate a dangerous set of conditions during the bypass procedure. Such drugs include: trimethaphan (Arfonad), and sodium nitroprusside (Nipride).

ANTI-ARRHYTHMIC DRUGS

The patient who experiences arrhythmias when on partial cardiopulmonary bypass will have abnormal ventricular ejections despite appropriate filling pressures. Propranolol is sometimes administered to patients with hypertrophied ventricles just prior to inducing hypothermia which permits myocardial cooling to the low 20° C range prior to aortic cross-clamping and administration of cardioplegia. Lidocaine (Xylocaine) is often given in the period after aortic cross- clamp removal when the cardiac rhythm is returning to normal and the patient is being rewarmed.

Anti-arrhythmic drugs should be administered into the bypass circuit on a physician's order, or by protocol, but will have little influence on perfusion technique.

CALCIUM ION ANTAGONISTS

The patient who comes to surgery for aortocoronary bypass graft surgery may be on calcium ion antagonists such as verapamil (Isoptin), diltiazem (Cardizem), or nifedipene (Procardia). These drugs sometimes are used in cardioplegic solutions, but do not affect cardiopulmonary bypass techniques as such. These drugs include: verapamil (Isoptin; Calan), and nifedipine (Procardia).

ANESTHETIC AGENTS

Nitrous oxide, if administered, should be turned off at least ten minutes prior to beginning cardiopulmonary bypass because of its theoretical capability of causing growth of gaseous microemboli.[12,13]

Other inhalational anesthetic agents are sometimes administered to the patient through the bypass circuit directly via the oxygenating gas to the oxygenator. The first effect on cardiopulmonary bypass could be the possible disintegration of the oxygenator or any other polycarbonate components of the bypass circuit should these agents be accidentally spilled on them.[14,15] Needless to say, the effect can be catastrophic since the time of disintegration is uncertain and the perfusionist may not be aware of the spillage.

The second concern with this technique is that an untrained person, the perfusionist, is "in control" of the anesthetic administration device. Communication between the anesthesiologist and perfusionist regarding the administration of such agents using this technique are of paramount importance. In higher concentrations, these gases can depress the myocardium, and many cases of inadequate or depressed hemodynamics have occurred because everyone "forgot" the anesthetic gas was still on at the pump. This oversight may be particularly common when on partial bypass and weaning the patient from bypass. Quite often the anesthesiologist is administering an inhalational anesthetic at the head of the table and the patient is therefore receiving twice the expected dose.

Other than a slight vasodilatory effect, properly used anesthetic agents do not affect cardiopulmonary bypass techniques.

ADJUNCTS TO ANESTHESIA

Muscle relaxants such as pancuronium bromide (Pavulon) or d-tubocurarie (Tubocurarine) are often administered during bypass to prevent patient movement or shivering. Both activities, if untreated, will increase oxygen consumption on bypass and may necessitate higher than expected flows. Patients given fentanyl (Sublimaze) and droperidol (Inapsine) together (Innovar) may exhibit slightly higher than normal perfusion pressures on bypass, but these drugs do not directly affect cardiopulmonary bypass techniques.

Dantrolene sodium (Dantrium) is given to counteract the metabolic disorder known as malignant hyperpyrexia or malignant hyperthermia. If a patient on bypass exhibits this life-threatening reaction, administration of Dantrolene plus perfusion hypothermia to 36° C will decrease oxygen consumption which may allow lower perfusion flow rates (see Chapter 19: EXISTING PATHOLOGY).

Thiopental sodium (Pentothal Sodium) has recently been advocated to decrease the incidence of neurologic dysfunction following cardiopulmonary bypass.[16] This drug causes severe hypotension at the dosages required for cerebral protection. Other than this effect and also prolonging the bypass time during weaning while vasopressors are given, administration of pentothal does not affect cardiopulmonary bypass techniques.

Antihistamines, sedative and narcotic agents, and non-narcotic pain medications are often given during open-heart surgery but none affect cardiopulmonary bypass techniques.

DIURETICS

Mannitol may be included in the pump prime according to protocol. Furosemide (Lasix) or ethacrynic acid (Edecrin) may be administered during cardiopulmonary bypass if urine output is decreased. Other than increasing fluid requirements if excessive diuresis occurs, these drugs do not affect cardiopulmonary bypass techniques.

ALKALYZING AGENTS

The ubiquitous sodium bicarbonate is used to counteract metabolic acidosis, a rare occurrence in clinical perfusion today. Sodium bicarbonate or Tris-hydroxy-methyl aminomethane (THAM) are frequently given with bank blood to raise the pH. Rarely, but quite effectively, sodium bicarbonate is given to reduce peripheral resistance. These drugs may slightly reduce venous return, but they do not affect cardiopulmonary bypass techniques.

STEROIDS

Methylprednisolone sodium succinate (Solu-Medrol) is sometimes given to small infants prebypass according to protocol. Cardiac transplantation patients also receive steroids, and steroids are used in the treatment of arterial air embolic events. The use of steroids does not affect cardiopulmonary bypass.

ANTIDIABETIC AGENTS

Insulin or oral antidiabetic drugs do not affect cardiopulmonary bypass techniques directly. One cautionary note however should be made regarding NPH insulin which contains minute quantities of protamine. Some patients have developed severe anaphalactic-type reactions following cardiopulmonary bypass when the heparin was reversed with protamine sulfate.[17] Therefore, diabetic patients who are on NPH insulin therapy should be watched carefully until it is determined that they have tolerated the protamine.

The perfusionist should be ready to restart cardiopulmonary bypass immediately if the patient's hemodynamics deteriorate to life-threatening levels. It is also worth noting that apparently the act of re-heparinizing the patient in anticipation of reinstituting bypass may ameliorate the protamine sensitivity effects by eliminating the action of the heparin-protamine complex.[18]

PERIPHERAL VASODILATORS

Patients who have been receiving IV nitroglycerin (Nitrostat, Nitro-Bid, Nitrol) sometimes exhibit heparin resistance,[19] which will not alter cardiopulmonary bypass techniques per se, but may necessitate higher than usual dosages of heparin and more frequent ACT measurements. Another recently reported consequences of IV nitroglycerin therapy is methemoglobinemia.[20-22] The blood during cardiopulmonary bypass will appear deeply cyanotic with paradoxically abnormally low oxygen saturation and normal pO_2s by arterial blood gas analysis. Treatment is administration of methylene blue and packed red blood cells. Technique considerations include use of a venous inline oxygen saturation sensor for early detection, and correction of metabolic acidosis that may have developed due to hypoperfusion. Papaverine hydrochloride sometimes is given to treat vascular spasm or more specifically to dilate the internal mammary artery prior to anastomosis during aortocoronary bypass graft operations. This drug does not affect bypass techniques.

SUMMARY

Cardiopulmonary bypass techniques are only minimally affected by pharmacologic therapy by the physician members of the open-heart surgery team. Simply an awareness of those few drugs that possibly may affect the conduct of perfusion is the most important cardiopulmonary bypass technique related to pharmacology.

REFERENCES

1. Cooper JB, Newbower RS, Kitz RJ: An analysis of major errors and equipment failures in anesthesia management: Considerations for prevention and detection. Anesthesiol 60:34, 1984.

2. Keenan RL, Boyan CP: Cardiac arrest due to anesthesia; A study of incidence and causes. JAMA 253:2373, 1985.
3. Bull BS, Huse WM, Brauer FS, Korpman RA: Heparin therapy during extracorporeal circulation.II. The use of a dose-response curve to individualize heparin and protamine dosage. J Thorac Cardiovasc Surg 69:685, 1975.
4. Freisen RH, Clement AJ: Individual responses to heparinization for extracorporeal circulation. J Thorac Cardiovasc Surg 72:875, 1976.
5. Kurusz M, Schneider B, Brown JP, Conti VR: Filtration during open-heart surgery: Devices, techniques, opinions and complications. Proceed Am Acad Cardiovasc Perfusion 4:123, 1983.
6. Bull BS, Korpman RA, Bull MH: Reply to Arkin CF, Shahsavari M, Copeland BE, Kim A: Evaluation of the activated clotting time to control heparin and protamine dosage in open-heart surgery (Letter to the Editor). J Thorac Cardiovasc Surg 75:790, 1978.
7. Smith JP, Walls JT, Muscato MS, McCord ES, Worth ER, Curtis JJ, Silver D: Extracorporeal circulation in a patient with heparin-induced thrombocytopenia. Anesthesiol 62:363, 1985.
8. Kakkasseril JB, Cranley JJ, Panke T, Grannan K: Heparin-induced thrombocytopenia: A prospective study of 142 patients. J Vasc Surg 2:382, 1985.
9. Olinger GN, Hussey CV, Olive JA, Malik MI: Cardiopulmonary bypass for patients with previously documented heparin-induced platelet aggregation. J Thorac Cardiovasc Surg 87:673, 1984.
10. Mabry CD, Read RC, Thompson BW, Williams CD, White HJ: Identification of heparin resistance during cardiac and vascular surgery. Arch Surg 114:129, 1979.
11. Esposito RA, Culliford AT, Colvin SB, Thomas SJ, Lackner H, Spencer FC: Heparin resistance during cardiopulmonary bypass; The role of heparin pretreatment. J Thorac Cardiovasc Surg 85:346, 1983.
12. Munson ES: Transfer of nitrous oxide into body air cavities. Br J Anaesth 46:202, 1974.
13. Bethune DW: Organ damage after open-heart surgery. Lancet 2:1410, 1976.
14. Maltry DE, Eggers Jr GWN: Isoflurane-induced failure of the Bentley-10 oxygenator (Letter). Anesthesiol 66:100, 1987.
15. Cooper S, Levin R: Near catastrophic oxygenator failure (Letter). Anesthesiol 66:101, 1987.
16. Nussmeir NA, Arlund C, Slogoff S: Neuropsychiatric complications after cardiopulmonary bypass: Cerebral protection by a barbiturate. Anesthesiol 64:155, 1986.
17. Kurusz M, Grant JA, Cooper JR, Conti VR, Arens JF: Protamine reactions in insulin-dependent diabetics following cardiopulmonary bypass. Proceed Am Acad Cardiovasc Perfusion 5:153, 1985.
18. Utley JR, Bhatt MA, Stephens DB, Kelley Jr HG: Reversal of protamine reaction with heparin. Perfusion 1:63, 1986.
19. Habbab MA, Haft JI: Heparin resistance induced by intravenous nitroglycerin; A word of caution when both drugs are used concomitantly. Arch Intern Med 147:857, 1987.
20. Armstrong D, Schmalfuss V, Reed CC, Stafford TB, McInnis RJ, Thompson DJ: A case study: Methemoglobinemia during cardiopulmonary bypass. Proceed Am Acad Cardiovasc Perfusion 6:179, 1985.
21. Robiscek F: Acute methemoglobinemia during cardiopulmonary bypass caused by intravenous nitroglycerin infusion. J Thorac Cardiovasc Surg 90:901, 1985
22. Bojar RM, Rastegar H, Payne DD, Harkness SH, England MR, Stetz JJ, Weiner B, Cleveland RJ: Methemoglobinemia from intravenous nitroglycerin: A word of caution Ann Thorac Surg 43:332, 1987.

..LAWSUITS AND ...CASENOTES

... During open-heart surgery for aortic valve replacement in a patient with severe calcific aortic stenosis, and prior to cannulation, the anesthesiologist administered what he thought was heparin. The heart was observed to go in to profound contracture ("Stone Heart"). Resuscitation was unsuccessful and the patient expired on the operating table. Investigation revealed that the patient had been injected with calcium by mistake.

... During an exceedingly long cardiopulmonary bypass procedure the serum potassium level rose to 6.0 mEq/L. When attempts were made to terminate bypass the heart was flabby and unable to produce an effective arterial pressure. The cardiac rhythm was complete heart block. The patient was unable to be weaned from cardiopulmonary bypass. The anesthesiologist administered one ampule of sodium bicarbonate, 10 USP units of insulin, and 50 ml of 50% Dextrose solution directly into the oxygenator. After five minutes of continued bypass the pharmacologic treatment was successful in driving potassium intra-cellularly. The patient converted to first degree heart block and the cardiac output was satisfactory. The patient was weaned from cardiopulmonary bypass without further incident.

Chapter 18:

MYOCARDIAL PROTECTION

Chapter 18: MYOCARDIAL PROTECTION

Myocardial protection is the one clear concise aspect of total cardiopulmonary bypass which fills the definition of circus movement.[1] Potassium cardioplegia was worked out completely in principle in 1958 and abandoned in 1960. Since its recent rediscovery, cardioplegia has become the hot buzz word topic and controversy. Current reports in the literature range from a series in which no cardioplegia was used[2] to the other end of the spectrum with the recent release of a commercially available cannula which resembles an octopus and the proposition of continuous infusion of cardioplegic solution of each separate graft as the proximal anastomosis is completed.[3]

The first attempts at myocardial protection were a sort of, "Oh, by the way" happening of total body hypothermia. Then coronary perfusion was practiced for many years on long cases, particularly aortic and double valve replacement. Coronary perfusion involved separate cannulation of both coronary arteries, and separate roller pumps, pressure monitors, and reservoirs to perfuse oxygenated mixed crystalloid and blood solution. The perfusionist who successfully perfused the aortic valve replacement with this technique was somewhat exhausted at the conclusion of the operation, but possessed a sense of real accomplishment. They were formidible cases from a technical standpoint.

Some centers used differential hypothermia in the coronary perfusion circuit, and the perfusate temperature was lowered to the range of 10-20° C. Many variations on this theme existed in the different open-heart centers.

Other centers continued the evolution, abandoning for the second time the technique of total body hypothermia. Myocardial protection now was achieved by anoxic arrest by cross-clamping the aorta and the technical speed of the surgeon. This was satisfactory until the "Stone Heart Syndrome" was described.[4]

Investigators turned back to hypothermia in the form of topical cooling, including the application of saline ice chips. Then the infusion of cold crystalloid in the aortic root was used. Finally, the surgeons rediscovered potassium cardioplegia, combined it with cold, added blood, then oxygenated the blood, finally adding a separate infusion pump with inline perfusion pressure monitor. To these authors, the only thing apparently left to do is to cannulate the separate coronary arteries and this has been done recently in the form of hand-held, rigid, disposable, coronary perfusion cannulae which, not surprisingly, closely resemble the stainless steel ones manufactured by Sarns, Inc. in the mid-1960s.

Comparative outcome studies are woefully lacking in the area of cardioplegia despite the amazing mass of publications on the subject. Perhaps we rush to embrace new techniques **only because they are new techniques** and appear logical in the absence of definitive outcome studies. To follow through with current thinking, in using the octopus catheter correctly one should monitor the pressure and flow in each cannula separately, thus during a 5 vessel graft procedure the perfusionist has 5 pressure monitors and 5 flows to watch *in addition to the oxygenator*, a practical impossibility and a grossly unsafe practice even in the attempt. If myocardial and/or graft damage can be caused by excessive pressure and flow, then these parameters should be measured during cardioplegia infusion (see Chapter 12: MONITORING). These authors believe the opportunity for kinking, malposition, and other mishaps leading to damage of the myocardium and/or grafts is greater when using such a device. If selective pressure and flow monitoring is not necessary and only flow and pressure monitoring into one end of the octopus cannula is required, because the flow and pressure will autoregulate itself, then perfusion retrograde through the coronary sinus would accomplish the same thing and in the same way. Additionally, retrograde perfusion would perfuse those distal coronary branches which have not yet been grafted. Retrograde coronary perfusion was first described and proposed in 1956.[5]

The proposition of oxygenated cold blood cardioplegia presents yet another somewhat confused technique. Below 10-15° C oxygen is so tightly bound to the blood that it essentially does not transport oxygen into the myocardium, other than that oxygen dissolved in plasma. Oxygenated crystalloid will supply as much or more oxygen to the myocardium under similar circumstances. So, why bother to add oxygenated blood to the cardioplegia solution and then cool it to 10° C prior to infusion? These are but more of the confusions surrounding cardioplegia.

These authors believe that the administration of cardioplegic solution, of whatever type, should be handled by the anesthesiologist who is possibly underutilized during cardiopulmonary bypass. The second preference is administration of cardioplegia by a second perfusionist. It is clear from The Survey that **administration of cardioplegia by the primary perfusionist is hazardous.** This practice not only detracts the perfusionist from their primary duty (see Chapter 1: DUTIES AND RESPONSIBILITIES) but is the source of an additional hazard to the patient. *The second most frequently reported cause of air embolus to the patient from the cardiopulmonary bypass circuit is the cardioplegia system.*

It is certainly possible to assemble a safe cardioplegia delivery system. It would require all the safety features which should be incorporated in the arterial line, i.e., inline filter with

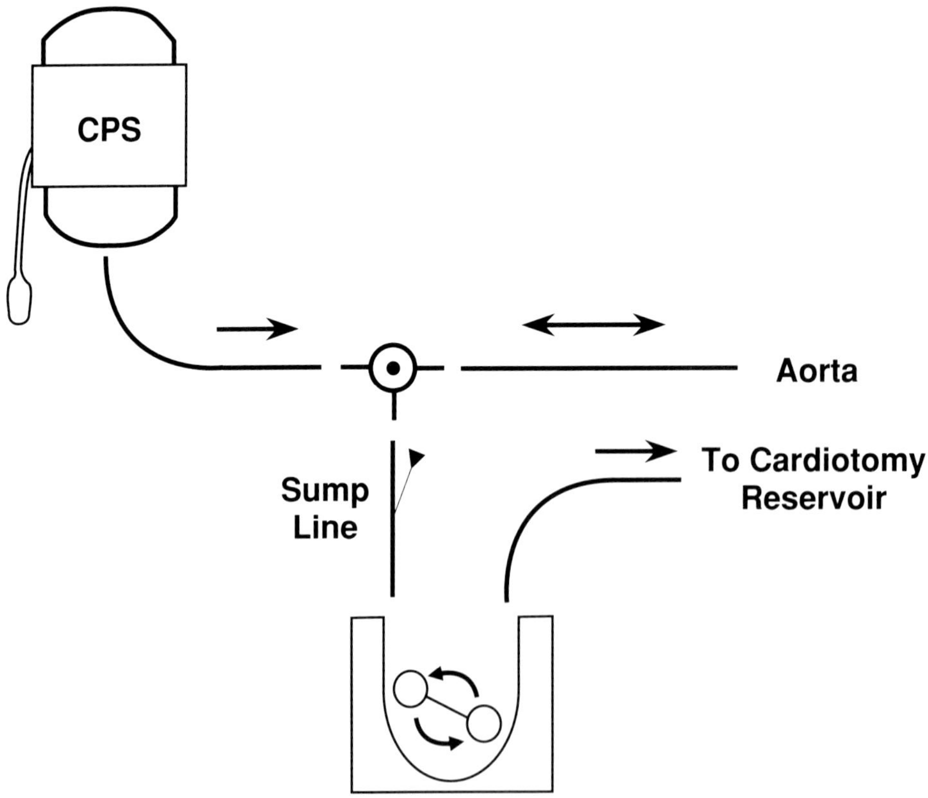

Figure 18.1 Diagram of the simple cardioplegia system utilizing the vent line and a stopcock for administration of cardioplegia solution from a pressurized IV administration bag. Note 25 gauge needle in sump line.

open purge line back to the oxygenator, bubble detector, pressure monitor, etc. The cost would seem to be prohibitive in today's environment. A second perfusionist or the anesthesiologist could provide a ready solution to the safe cardioplegia delivery system question. The controversy over the benefits of cardioplegia in the routine open-heart surgery procedure is more unclear and tumultuous than the question of arterial line filtration ever was.

The most convenient cardioplegia administration system is shown in Figure 18.1. Normally the anesthesiologist manages the IV administration set, bag, and pressure pump. The surgeon manipulates the three-way stopcock to either infuse cardioplegic solution or to start sumping/venting or to shut the system off. Blood cardioplegia can be administered through this system by using a Y type administration set and by placing blood in the second IV bag and mixing the two prior to administration. This system has the drawback of uncontrolled temperature. Normally the cardioplegic solution is taken from the refrigerator and administered immediately. Subsequent administrations from this set-up will not be at the same cold temperature as the first. Another problem with this system is the possibility of administration of air from excessive pressure on the IV bag and inattention of the adminis-

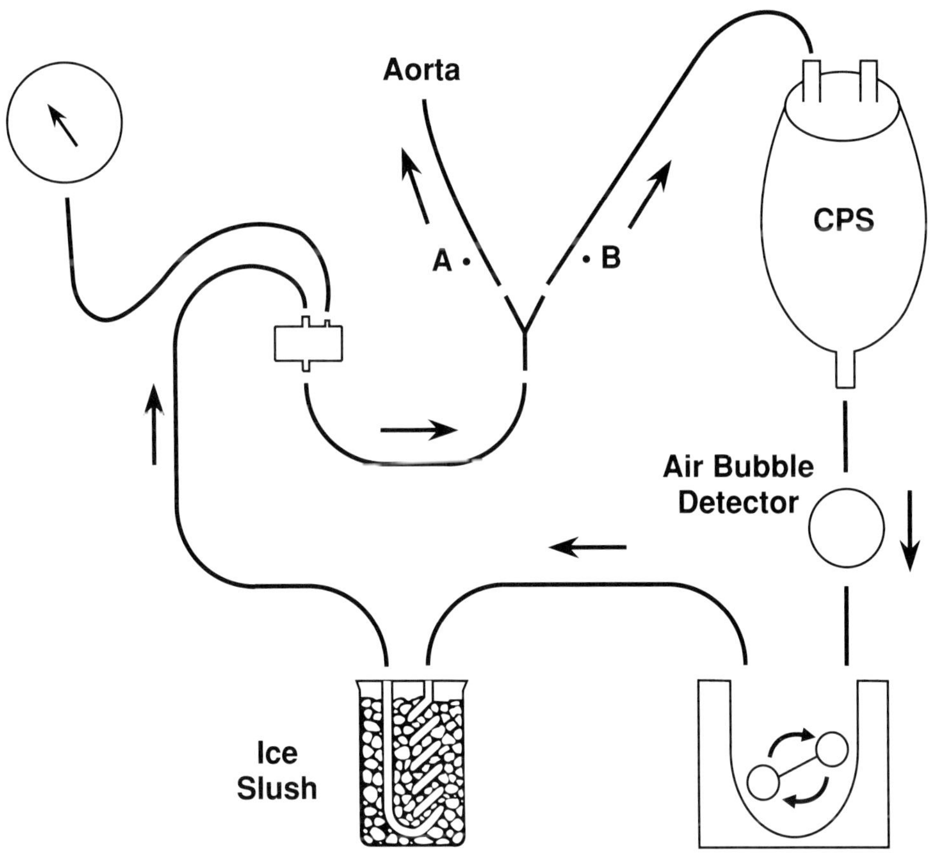

Figure 18.2 Recommended cardioplegia system incorporating such safety features as an inline filter, pressure gauge, and air bubble detector. By clamping the line at point A, continuous recirculation is possible maintaining cardioplegia temperature. By clamping the circuit at point B, cardioplegic solution is directed into the aorta. An inline filter constantly filters the cardioplegic solution.

trator. The possibility also exists that the surgeon may turn the stopcock the wrong way or that the stopcock will leak thus aspirating air into the system which may be pumped into the patient.

Figure 18.2 shows the recommended cardioplegia delivery system. A heat exchanger may be substituted for the ice bucket which will give more positive control over the temperature. A pressure monitor is also incorporated in the system to aid in avoiding overpressurization, and an air bubble detector is located between the cardioplegia reservoir and roller pump.

Most investigators believe an aortic root perfusion pressure of 60-100 mmHg should be maintained during cardioplegia administration, the implication being that flow rate or volume is of secondary importance. This seems a bit contradictory. The first goal of cardioplegia is to reduce the temperature of the myocardium. This is only accomplished by an adequate flow for a measurable time at a specific inward temperature. It seems more reasonable that pressure, at least as high as that found in the patient preoperation, along with a flow rate of 150-300 ml/min should be maintained. Coincidentally these are the parameters for the old coronary perfusion technique.

REFERENCES

1. Keats AS: The Rovenstine Lecture, 1983: Cardiovascular anesthesia: Perceptions and perspectives. Anesthesiology 60:467, 1984.
2. Bonchek LJ, Burlingame MW: Coronary bypass without cardioplegia. J Thorac Cardiovasc Surg 93:261, 1987.
3. Lawrie GM: A simple technique for multigraft cardioplegic infusion during coronary artery bypass. Ann Thorac Surg 39:483, 1985.
4. Cooley DA, Reul GJ, Wukasch DC: Ischemic contracture of the heart: "Stone Heart." Am J Cardiology 29:575, 1972.
5. Blanco G, Adam A, Fernandez A, Raffuci F: Direct experimental approach to the aortic valve, presented at the Sixth Annual Meeting of the Puerto Rico Chapter of the American College of Surgeons, San Juan, February, 1956.

..LAWSUITS AND ...CASENOTES

... During the administration of cardioplegic solution, the cardioplegia reservoir was emptied and air was aspirated into the aorta. Active infusion had been stopped, but air was sucked into the aorta through the vent line which was one of a multiple outlet cardioplegia set.

... One case of gas embolism due to cardioplegia administration with no injury.

... Two cases of gas embolism due to cardioplegia administration with one death and one permanent injury.

... Two cases of gas embolism due to cardioplegia administration with one permanent injury and one no injury.

... Blood for a blood cardioplegia system was being drawn from a Y in the arterial line. The blood was allowed to travel part way up to the blood cardioplegia reservoir and then the line was clamped. Inadvertently, the reservoir was pressurized and when the clamp was removed to completely fill the line to the reservoir, air was forced backwards into the arterial line and into the patient. There was no injury.

... Towards the end of bypass the blood cardioplegia fluid remaining in the cardioplegia reservoir was being returned to the bypass circuit retrograde through a Y in the arterial line. Air was pumped into the arterial line. The constantly purging arterial line filter worked properly, and the air was purged back to the oxygenator. No patient injury occurred.

... During aortocoronary bypass graft surgery the surgeon noticed air bubbling out of the coronary arteriotomy. The entire cardioplegia system was free of fluid and was actively pumping air into the aortic root. Routine deairing of the heart was carried out. At the time the arterial pump was stopped, air rose up into the aortic cannula. No patient injury was reported.

Chapter 19:

EFFECTS OF EXISTING PATHOLOGY ON CARDIOPULMONARY BYPASS

Chapter 19: EFFECTS OF EXISTING PATHOLOGY ON CARDIOPULMONARY BYPASS

Existing patient pathology may or may not have an effect on cardiopulmonary bypass. If it has been diagnosed or anticipated, existing pathology should not be a problem to the perfusionist or to the bypass procedure. If it is undiagnosed, preexisting pathology can present the open-heart team problems approaching emergency proportions. As always, the perfusionist should be prepared for any eventuality in the patient, the bypass equipment, or the operating room.

ATHEROSCLEROSIS

Eighty to ninety per cent of the cardiopulmonary bypass procedures involve aortocoronary bypass graft surgery. Coronary artery disease is a manifestation of atherosclerosis in the coronary arteries. If this disease is present in these vessels it is logical to assume that the disease is widespread throughout the body. Consequently cerebrovascular disease and/or carotid artery occlusive disease may also be present.

In the presence of either of the other two disease entities or if their presence is suspected, the perfusion pressure should be increased accordingly. A useful guide is the patient's pre-surgical blood pressure record. If a perfusion pressure of 50-60 mmHg is considered normal for a patient whose normal pressure is 120-130/80-90 mmHg then a perfusion pressure for a patient with a record of 140-160/80-90 mmHg should be 60-70 mmHg. This is not a decision that should be made solely by the perfusionist, but in consultation with the anesthesiologist and the surgeon if not specifically addressed in the protocol.

Patients with concomitant coronary artery disease and an abdominal aneurysm may be operated on in two stages. The heart is revascularized prior to a second operation to repair the aneurysm. In these cases bypass is performed in the same fashion as for a routine case. Retrograde perfusion with femoral cannulation is contraindicated.

If the aorta appears to be diseased at palpation by the surgeon, serious consideration should be given to inserting the arterial cannula into the femoral artery and perfusing the patient retrograde. In the presence of severe disease of the aorta cross-clamping can be avoided entirely, but the amount of suction blood will be increased significantly. Very small tip suckers can be used and will keep the field of the distal anastomosis relatively clear. If further hemostasis is necessary, digital pressure can be applied proximal to the anastomosis site. These considerations are, of course, surgical in nature, but are included because of their implications for cardiopulmonary bypass.

THE ANEPHRIC OR ANEURIC PATIENT

The absence of kidneys or renal function is no contraindication for cardiopulmonary bypass. With today's technology cardiopulmonary bypass should be carried out in normal fashion utilizing routine protocols. Priming solutions should be limited to those which contain less than 5 mEq/L of potassium. Potassium cardioplegia should be avoided but many cases have and are being done with only topical hypothermia. Hemodialysis can be carried out the day or evening before surgery, as soon as the patient is transported to the recovery room, or during cardiopulmonary bypass itself. The dialysate can easily be customized to the particular needs of the individual patient. The Nephrologist will need to know what drugs and solutions the patient received, or will receive in the operating room, in order to customize the dialysate for either dialysis location.

If the decision is made to dialyze the patient during bypass the only additional equipment needed is a Y connector in the arterial line proximal to the arterial line filter and sufficient tubing and reducers to connect this line to the dialyzer cartridge and return it to the cardiotomy reservoir. The arterial flow rate should be increased to compensate for the volume being diverted through the dialyzer, which is usually in the order of 300 ml/min (see Figure 7.1).

While the hemoconcentrator only removes water by the process of ultrafiltration, using pressure to squeeze water across the semipermeable membrane, a dialysis cartridge removes any chemicals or ions which are in a higher concentration in the blood than they are in the dialysate fluid. Pressure is used in the process but it is negative pressure on the dialysate fluid side of the microcapillary membranes. If, for example, the K^+ concentration in the dialysate fluid is 3.9 then the blood is dialyzed against this value and the K^+ concentration of the blood cannot go below 3.9. The dialysate fluid can be tailor made, as far as the chemicals and ions are concerned, for the individual patient.

THE PREGNANT PATIENT

Total cardiopulmonary bypass in the pregnant patient has been on the increase in recent years, and with proper monitoring and perfusion techniques along with successful surgery there is no reason for mother and infant not to do well postoperatively. A large percent of the cases reported involve patients with Marfan's syndrome. Because of surgical anatomy, arterial return is to the left femoral artery. This perhaps is the proper location to cannulate all pregnant patients. With this set-up the uterine and placental arteries are supplied with blood at the highest oxygen content provided for the patient. Atrial cannulation is via the right atrium.

A fetal monitor must be used during the entire bypass procedure, and it is advisable to have an Obstetrician observing the monitor and advising the perfusionist. Fetal distress is readily apparent on the fetal monitor. Fetal distress is directly related to perfusion flow. Bypass should be started at a calculated blood flow rate of 70-80 ml/kg/min or 2.6-3.0 L/min/m^2. The flow can then be adjusted up or down as the fetal monitor dictates. As stated, fetal distress is directly and almost instantaneously related to blood flow rate.

Beyond the techniques mentioned above, cardiopulmonary bypass should be conducted as usual. The effects of hypothermia on the fetus has not yet been clearly defined. Successful cases have been reported with normothermia and with hypothermia to 20°C. ACTs should be monitored every 20 minutes and adjusted as necessary.

PERSISTENT LEFT SUPERIOR VENA CAVA

Persistent left superior vena cava is most frequently an autopsy finding. It causes no problem to the patient, only to the cardiac surgeon and only if the right heart is opened. With single atrial cannulation blood return from the three cavae is provided for. If the right heart is opened, blood return from the left superior vena cava may obscure the surgeon's view of the operative field, but this may be cleared with a third sucker or by direct intra-cardiac cannulation. If intra-cardiac cannulation is employed, the three caval cannulae should be of the same length from the proximal Y connector to the distal tips of the three cannulae (see Figure 19.1).

Bypass is normal except for the cannulation techniques. If the third cava is not cannulated and the right heart is opened the perfusionist should be prepared for significant suction return and a third sucker is sometimes of great benefit.

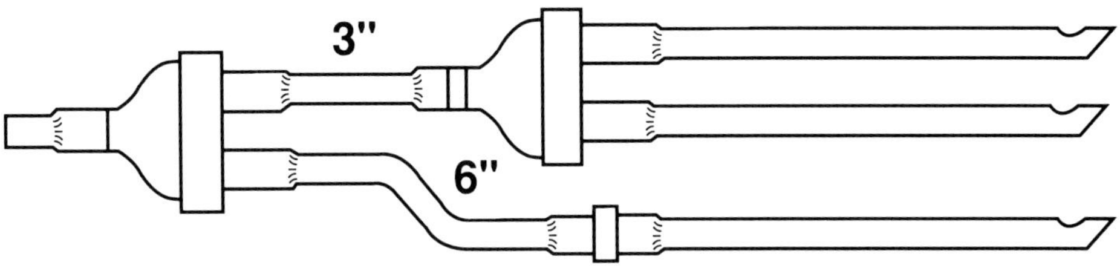

Figure 19.1 Shows the three caval cannulae set-up for use in a persistent left superior vena cava. Note that the ends of the cannulae are equidistant from the venous line connector.

VSD WITH UNDIAGNOSED PATENT DUCTUS ARTERIOSUS

If not discovered prior to surgery, many times the perfusionist is the first to diagnose the patent ductus arteriosus. Once the VSD has been repaired the venous return diminishes dramatically as the lungs become engorged with blood. Flow should be reduced to prevent pulmonary edema and the surgeon notified immediately of the situation and the suspected undiagnosed pathology.

PALLIATIVE SHUNT

The presence of a Potts shunt, Cooley shunt, or other type palliative type shunt presents a temporary inconvenience and challenge to the perfusionist. When bypass is commenced the venous return will be much less than anticipated or calculated. Increasing arterial blood flow will only increase the perfusion problem.

The shunt diverts arterial blood to the lungs and increasing arterial flow simply shunts more and more blood to the lungs. The perfusionist finds himself perfusing in a circle and increasing the flow beyond a certain volume will only increase the speed with which the blood transits the inter-thoracic circle. Caution must be exercised or profound pulmonary edema can result from overperfusion.

Perfusion with this preexisting pathology must be carried out with patience. The team must balance arterial flow with shunt flow, increasing arterial blood flow as high as possible without shunting too much flow to the capillary beds of the lungs.

Once the shunt has been taken down or clamped, normal venous return may be expected and the remainder of the case should proceed in a normal fashion.

MYXOMA AND MURAL THROMBUS

During removal of an atrial myxoma or resection of a ventricular aneurysm with mural thrombus and rarely even with a calcific aortic valve resection, the perfusionist is presented with another set of problems which should be anticipated. Sometimes so much clot, debris, or tissue is recovered through the suction system that it clots the cardiotomy reservoir. This is particularly true with cardiotomy reservoirs with integral filters (see Chapter 8: FILTRATION).

At other times it appears that the debris itself does not occlude the reservoir by volume but rather initiates coagulation within the reservoir. When this occurs the cardiotomy and extracorporeal filter must be changed. If possible the blood contained in the system should be washed and filtered before being returned to the bypass circuit and patient. When this is not possible, filtration is mandatory and a combination screen and depth type filter is preferable.

Right atrial myxomas may also embolize to the oxygenator through the venous line, especially with the single two-stage atrial cannulation technique.

BIBLIOGRAPHY FOR PERFUSION DURING PREGNANCY

Bahery CM, Ninio A, Gorodesky IG, Neri A: Toco cardiography in pregnancy during extracorporeal bypass for mitral valve replacement. Isr J Med Sci 16:359, 1980.

Bigley J, Reed CC, Thompson D, Stafford TB, McInnis RJ, Berryessa R:Repair of ascending aortic aneurysm in a pregnant patient with Marfan's syndrome: A case report. Proceed Amer Acad Cardiovas Perfusion 6:191, 1985.

Collins HA, Daniel RA, Scott HW: Cardiac surgery during pregnancy. Ann Thorac Surg 5:300, 1968.

Cohn LH, Shumway NE: Pulmonary embolectomy during pregnancy. Arch Surg 106:214, 1973.

Dubourg G, Broustet P: Complete correction of Fallot's triad in extracorporeal circulation. Arch Mal Coeur 52:1389, 1959.

Eilen B, Kaiser IH, Becker RM, Cohn MN: Aortic valve replacement during the third trimester of pregnancy. Obstet Gynecol 57:119, 1981.

Halseth WL, Elliot DP, Walker EL, Smith EA: Open mitral commissurotomy. J Thorac Cardiovasc Surg 80:842, 1980.

Harthorne JW, Buckly MJ, Grover JW, Austen WG: Valve replacement during pregnancy. Ann Intern Med 67:1032, 1967.

Jacobs WM, Cooley DA, Goen GP: Cardiac surgery with extracorporeal circulation during pregnancy. Obstet Gynecol 25:167, 1965.

Kay CF, Smith D: Surgery in the pregnant cardiac patient. Am J Cardiol 12:293, 1963.

Koh KS, Friesen RM, Livingstone RA, Peddle LJ: Fetal monitoring during maternal cardiac surgery with cardiopulmonary bypass. Canad Med Assoc J 112:1402, 1975.

Kozam RL, Conklin EF, Giannelli S, Serey P, Chu D: Open-heart for surgery mitral stenosis during pregnancy. J Thorac Cardivasc Surgery 53:587, 1967.

Lamp MP, Rass K, Kohnstone AM, Mannrs JM: Fetal heart monitoring during open-heart surgery. Br J Obstet Gynaecol 88:669, 1981.

Lee Jr WH, Pate JW: Surgical aspect of heart disease in pregnancy. GP 28:78, 1963.

Lyse R, Ofstun M, Dillard DH, Merendino KA: Congenital aortic stenosis in pregnancy, corrected by extracorporeal circulation. JAMA 176:1009, 1961.

Mannix EP, Mahajan DR: Open-heart surgery during pregnancy; A report of three cases. J Thorac Cardiovasc Surg 53:592,1967.

Marcinkevicius A, et al: Pulmonary embolectomy during pregnancy. J Cardiovasc Surg 11:355, 1970.

Martin MC, Pernoll ML, Boruszak AN, et al: Cesarean section while on cardiac bypass: Report of a case. Obstet Gynecol 57: 415, 1981.

Meffert WG, Stansel HG: Open-heart surgery during pregnancy. Am J Obstet Gynecol 102:1116, 1968.

Page PA: Cardiopulmonary bypass combined with fetal monitoring for removal of a left atrial myxoma during pregnancy. JECT 13:167, 1981.

Robinson M, Newman N, Creevy DC, Katz J, Harrison DC: Congenital aortic stenosis in pregnancy. JAMA 200:108, 1967.

Roe BB, Edmunds LH, Fishman NH, Hutchinson JC: Open mitral valvulotomy. Ann Thorac Surg 12:483, 1971.

Trimakas AP, Maxwell KD, Berkaky S, et al: Fetal monitoring during cardiopulmonary bypass for removal of a left atrial myxoma during pregnancy. Johns Hopkins Med J 144:156, 1979.

Werch A, Lambert HM, Cooley D: Fetal monitoring and maternal open-heart surgery. Southern Med J 70:1024, 1977.

Wright DM, Malloy KP, Reed CC: Cardiopulmonary perfusion of a patient with Marfan's syndrome with an associated ascending aortic aneurysm and an undiagnosed atrial septal defect. Proceed Amer Acad Cardiovasc Perfusion 2:86, 1981.

Zitnik RS, Brandenburg RO, Sheldon R, et al: Pregnancy and open-heart surgery. Circulation 39:257, 1969.

Zuhdi N, Carey J, Schmidt A, Greer A: Total body perfusion and pregnancy. J Int Coll Surg 43:43, 1965.

..LAWSUITS AND ...CASENOTES

... Shortly after going on complete bypass the perfusionist received the first blood gas analysis. The pO_2 was 300 mmHg. The oxygenator was examined and the blood appeared a sort of "chocolate brown color." A stat blood sample was sent to the clinical laboratory for analysis for methemoglobin. The results were positive, methylene blue was given, and bypass continued uneventfully.

Chapter 20:

EFFECTS OF SURGICAL TECHNIQUE ON CARDIOPULMONARY BYPASS

Chapter 20: EFFECTS OF SURGICAL TECHNIQUE ON CARDIOPULMONARY BYPASS

The techniques utilized by the primary surgeon and the manipulations he performs can have direct effects on cardiopulmonary bypass. In the worst case these effects can be catastrophic in nature, and even more so if the perfusionist is blissfully unaware of what is happening at the operating field and communication between the teams is less than effective (see Chapter 3: INTERFACE).

SINGLE ATRIAL CANNULATION

Perhaps the surgical technique that has the most profound effect on cardiopulmonary bypass is single atrial cannulation. The technique itself has been previously described as "the open manhole cover method of perfusion."[1] A single, large bore, usually 52 French, cannula is inserted into the right atrium. The cannula may be two-staged, that is be of two different diameters with holes at the distal end and another set of holes where the two sizes of tubing meet, or may be of one diameter throughout the entire length with a set of holes in the distal end and another set of holes two inches back. The theory is that the distal tip is inserted into the inferior vena cava and drains blood from that area while the proximal set of holes drains all blood entering the right atrium. This technique is particularly appealing for aortocoronary bypass graft procedures.

If this cannulation technique is employed by the surgeon, total cardiopulmonary bypass is not possible in the classic sense. All the blood returning through the superior and inferior cavae is no longer directed through the venous line. It is possible for blood to bypass the venous line and continue on into the pulmonary circulation. During manipulation of the heart the venous return is not protected by separate cannulae with this technique, and the incidence of caval obstruction, superior caval congestion, cerebral congestion, and diminished venous return is increased. It is mandatory that loss of venous return be communicated *immediately* to the surgeon and anesthesiologist. The anesthesiologist can check the patient for signs of superior caval obstruction or congestion.

Attempts to translocate volume, or to hold up volume in the patient, floods the operating field with blood. Using this cannulation technique essentially eliminates any effect on pressure the perfusionist may have since he can neither increase flows nor shift volumes. Resultant perfusion pressures are usually below those normally experienced or expected.

If the patient has an undiagnosed atrial septal defect or patent foramen ovale and the left heart is opened, the air lock in the venous line is sudden, abrupt, and total. All venous return is lost until the defect is repaired since the source of the air lock is still present.

Using this technique seems to increase the number of venous air locks and auto-decannulations. Perhaps, if the technique of retrograde cardioplegia infusion through the coronary sinus proves to be the technique of choice, single atrial cannulation will be relegated to the history books.

MALPOSITION OF CANNULA

Malposition of the venous cannula/ae usually affects the venous return during bypass. Venous return is diminished and will remain so until the cannulae are repositioned. This is sometimes diagnosed by the anesthesiologist from observing right-sided head and/or neck congestion. Cerebral congestion and edema can occur if the condition is not corrected.

Malposition of the arterial cannula manifests itself to the perfusionist as increasing arterial line pressure which is most often abrupt, but may be gradual in occurring. If aortic dissection occurs due to the malposition, the increase in arterial pressure in this situation is instantaneous and usually extremely high. A sudden increase or increasing arterial line pressure should be communicated to the surgeon immediately.

Enthusiastic retraction of the heart during bypass can result in cannula malposition but more frequently this maneuver simply kinks the venous cannula thus compromising venous return. The arterial cannula can also be kinked resulting in increased line pressure, parting of tubing and connectors, or rupture of the tubing itself.

If the innominate artery is inadvertently cannulated the result can include: engorgement of the arm and right carotid artery, increased arterial line pressure, diminished blood flow to the left carotid artery with resultant hypoperfusion to the left cerebral hemisphere. The right sided hyperperfusion can ultimately cause serous fluid to be observed leaking from the patient's ear. Prior to this generally fatal condition, the venous blood gases will have decreased along with increasing base deficits indicating that systemic perfusion is inadequate.

All of the possible emergencies and complications mentioned above have and continue to be reported with accompanying permanent injury or death of patients.

REOPERATION (REDO)

Reoperation with repeat median sternotomy and thoracotomy presents the perfusionist with a potential life-threatening emergency situation. It is not extraordinary for the surgeon to saw into the right ventricular cavity. Even if the chest is successfully opened, any other part of the myocardium, previous bypass grafts, or great vessels can be torn while spreading the sternum or dissecting the heart free from adhesions.[2]

The perfusionist must be prepared to go on bypass with only the suction system and be prepared with connectors and tubing to convert to femoral cannulation. Normally arterial return is to the femoral artery and venous return is through the suckers until right atrial cannulation can be accomplished. This is a perfectly safe perfusion technique and a completely survivable emergency.

ORDER OF ANASTOMOSES

Customarily during aortocoronary bypass grafting, the surgeon performs the distal anastomoses first on total cardiopulmonary bypass and the proximal anastomoses on partial bypass or off bypass with a partially occluding clamp. Some surgeons prefer to reverse this procedure and perform the proximal anastomoses first, off bypass with a partially occluding clamp if possible, or on partial bypass if necessary. The surgeon initiates total bypass and performs the distal anastomoses. With this technique, the graft must be clamped while being sewn in distally. Once the anastomoses is complete the clamp is removed and blood allowed to flow through the new graft. Suction return may be increased from the other anastomoses sites depending upon the anatomy of the myocardial circulation. Perfusion times are usually comparable and this technique presents no new or unusual problems for the perfusionist.

CRYOPRECIPITATE

The unannounced use of cryoprecipitate "fibrin glue" can have catastrophic effects on the cardiopulmonary bypass procedure. It is possible to clot the entire bypass circuit by unsuspectingly aspirating this drug through the suction system. Should this occur, the perfusionist has no choice but to stop bypass immediately and to set up another bypass circuit as rapidly as possible. Since this is a time-limited, life-threatening emergency, the perfusionist need only be concerned with setting up an oxygenator and an arterial and venous line. Suckers, vents, and a cardiotomy reservoir can be added after cardiopulmonary bypass has been reestablished.

CLAMPS

The application of any clamp by the surgeon or others at the operative field to any of the bypass lines without the knowledge of the perfusionist can have disastrous results. Sometimes, the application of a clamp to the patient's anatomy can have similar results. It is very important that the surgeon inform the perfusionist before applying any clamps to any of the bypass lines. It is equally important that the perfusionist be aware of anatomical clamping being performed by the surgeon.

REFERENCES

1. Reed CC: Total cardiopulmonary bypass fondly remembered. Proceed Am Acad Cardiovasc Perfusion 2:25, 1981.
2. Dobell ARC, Jain AK: Catastrophic hemorrhage during redo sternotomy. Ann Thorac Surg 37:273, 1984.

..LAWSUITS AND ...CASENOTES

.. At the end of bypass the surgeon, assistant surgeon, and anesthesiologist observed air rising in the arterial cannula. The surgeon informed the family that the perfusionist had pumped air into the patient. The patient died that evening. The family filed suit against the perfusionist, but the attorney refused to sue the surgeon. At trial the jury found in favor of the perfusionist defendant. The family then filed suit against the surgeon. At trial, the plaintiff held that the surgeon had not adequately de-aired the heart. The surgeon held that the perfusionist pumped air, even though an arterial line filter with open purge line was used in addition to a bubble detector and a low level alarm sensor. The jury was not allowed to know that the perfusionist had already been sued and found not negligent. The jury then found for the plaintiff surgeon thinking that the perfusionist was at fault. The family then sued the attorney for malpractice for not suing the surgeon in the first place. The case was settled out of court for an amount in excess of $225,000.

.. The surgeon inserted a right superior pulmonary vein vent without first testing the function of the vent and without cross-clamping the aorta. The perfusionist had reversed the vent and air was pumped into the patient. The patient died and suit was filed against the perfusionist, the hospital, and the surgeon. The jury found for the plaintiff in the amount of $750,000 holding that both the perfusionist and the surgeon were liable.

.. The surgeon inserted a left atrial vent through the right superior pulmonary vein and opened the left ventricle without first cross-clamping the aorta. The patient died. Suit was filed against the surgeon who then filed suit against the perfusionist. The jury awarded the plaintiff $650,000 finding the defendant surgeon liable.

... One open-heart team reported two cases of air embolus from stopcocks on the central venous pressure line being open to air. Venous air lock resulted in both cases with one resultant patient death.

... Two patient deaths reported in which the heart was not de-aired before the cross-clamp was removed and the heart began ejecting unexpectedly.

... The patient suffered air embolism and died. The cause was an open stopcock on the arterial cannula/arterial line connector when bypass began. Air was sucked in through the stopcock and pumped in the patient's arterial system.

... The surgeon inserted a vent catheter before cross-clamping the aorta, the heart beat and sucked air in through the vent and pumped the air out the aorta. The patient died.

... Air was pumped into the aorta via a pressure monitoring line after the completion of cardiopulmonary bypass. The patient died.

... During a total power failure during surgery and in total darkness the surgeon inadvertently removed the aortic cross-clamp while the left ventricle was open. The perfusionist was attempting to clamp the arterial line at the time. The patient died.

... Air embolus occurred while surgeon was making incision and prior to insertion of left heart vent. Aorta had not been cross-clamped and the heart was still beating. The patient died.

... Air embolus occurred while surgeon was inserting an unclamped vent line through the right superior pulmonary vein with a beating heart and uncross-clamped aorta. The patient died.

... At the termination of bypass air filled the aortic cannula retrograde from the aortic root. The cross-clamp was removed and the patient died on the second postoperative day.

... The surgeon was using a single atrial cannula and during bypass, the cannula backed out of the atrium to the point that the proximal holes in the cannula were outside the right atrium. A massive venous air embolus occurred and passed through the membrane oxygenator. There was no arterial line filter in use. The patient died.

... Single atrial cannulation was being used and the cannula auto-decannulated. A massive venous air-lock occurred, the arterial reservoir level was lost, and the patient suffered a massive air embolus. No arterial line filter was in use, no bubble detector or low level alarm sensors were in use. The patient died.

... During cardiopulmonary bypass a bored or distracted resident surgeon clamped the arterial line. The line separated at a slip connector and the results resembled a loose fire hose. The patient suffered no ill effects, but housekeeping personnel had to work overtime cleaning the blood off the ceiling, in the lights, air conditioning ducts, etc..

... After aortic cannulation and connection to the arterial line, the assistant surgeon towel clipped the arterial line to the side of the operating field and covered the line with a towel. Twenty-three minutes after bypass began the anesthesiologist noted emboli in the retinae of the patient. The bypass circuit was inspected with negative results. Finally the primary surgeon inspected the arterial cannula and its connection to the arterial line. It was discovered that the towel clamp had punctured line and that air had been sucked into the arterial line since the start of bypass. The patient did not survive.

... After replacement of the aortic valve and ascending aorta with a valved conduit prosthesis cryoprecipitate or "fibrin glue" was applied to the bleeding suture line while on cardiopulmonary bypass. The assistant surgeon continued using the pump suckers and the perfusionist was unaware that the drug had been utilized. The perfusionist noticed an uneven blood level in the oxygenator reservoir. Bypass was terminated uneventfully but during transfusion of the contents of the oxygenator massive blood clots were discovered. Transfusion was stopped immediately. The cardiotomy was also totally clotted. There was no apparent sequelae and the patient made an uneventful recovery.

... After connecting the arterial line to the aortic cannula, the surgeon observed air in the arterial line. Instead of disconnecting and reconnecting the arterial line, the surgeon inserted a 25 gauge needle three times through the arterial line to aspirate small gas bubbles. During the operation, the anesthesiologist noted gas infarcts in the patient's retinal arteries. The patient did not regain consciousness. Air was aspirated into the arterial line during the perfusion through the needle holes.

... When the surgeon applied the aortic cross-clamp the arterial pressure monitor "pegged out" at the maximum reading. The perfusionist stopped the pump, slowly reversed the pumphead until the line pressure had been reduced. The surgeon released the aortic cross-clamp, which had also clamped the end of the aortic cannula, and bypass was resumed. There was no apparent injury to the patient.

... The surgeon applied the aortic cross-clamp and the arterial cannula separated from the arterial line. The pump was stopped and the line reconnected to the cannula. The surgeon released the cross-clamp freeing the end of the aortic cannula, and bypass was resumed.

.. During aortocoronary bypass graft surgery, the surgeon kinked the venous return line, the perfusionist did not notice the falling reservoir level in time, and air vortexed into the arterial line with an arterial reservoir level of 200 ml. The air bubble detector worked effectively and stopped the arterial pumphead. At that point the surgeon "flashed" the aortic cross-clamp. The patient did not regain consciousness. The surviving family members filed suit against the surgeon. The case was settled out of court for an undisclosed amount.

... Historical note. Dr. Robert Liston, Scottish anatomist and surgeon of the mid-19th century, is the only physician to have a 300% mortality rate for a single operation. During a two-and-a-half minute amputation, the patient died in hospital from gangrene, he amputated the fingers of his young assistant, who died in hospital of gangrene, and slashed through the coattails of a surgical spectator, who thought that the knife had pierced his vitals, suffered a coronary, and dropped dead on the spot.

... For aortocoronary bypass grafting the aortic perfusion cannula was a beveled type inserted into the ascending aorta. Immediately after establishing total bypass, the mean arterial blood pressure increased from 95 to 110 mmHg with distinct 40 mmHg pulse pressure waves that coincided with the roller pump rotations. The arterial line pressure was normal. Halothane (3%) was used to treat the hypertension. One hour later, the left radial artery pressure was still 100 mmHg, but the patient's pupils were noted to be mid-size and non-reactive to light. Malposition of the arterial cannula was confirmed when the surgeon withdrew the cannula 3 cm, and the mean arterial pressure suddenly fell to normal values and the phasic waves diminished. Bypass was discontinued without difficulty and the patient had no neurologic sequelae.

Chapter 21:

AUTOTRANSFUSION

Chapter 21: AUTOTRANSFUSION

Autotransfusion was first reported by Blundell in 1818.[1] He was either afraid someone might have missed reading it the first time (see Figure 21.1), or was so enamoured with the idea that he published the technique again ten years later (see Figure 21.2).[2] Other citations have appeared infrequently in the literature. One hundred years passed before Elmendorf reported the first use of autotransfusion in a case of hemothorax using blood shed in the thoracic cavity of a soldier.[3] Reports sporadically have appeared in the literature in the years between these two reports and continue down to the present time including one successful case from the island of Samoa.[4-10] Lockwood was the first investigator to report its use in the United States.[5]

During the early 1970s there was renewed interest in autotransfusion.[11-14] The technique gained a measure of acceptance and success in the beginning. However, reports of accidents and iatrogenic disseminated intravascular coagulation (DIC) led to the abrupt general disappearance of the technique by the mid-to-late 1970s.[11-22]

The technique of autotransfusion is a sound technique in principle however. The problems experienced by early investigators stemmed from lack of knowledge of physiology (recall that heparin was not discovered until 1917), and by later investigators due to limitations of equipment and techniques. Added to this was the fact that autotransfusion systems were placed in small community hospitals where personnel were only superficially trained in the techniques, and the clinical laboratories were unable to assist in diagnosing post-usage clinical problems. It is yet another instance of medical irony that John Duncan of Edinburgh wrote in 1886 that his colleagues should not "neglect stringent precautions needful to avoid the contingencies of septicity and embolism, lest [autotransfusion] should fall into discredit from too wide an application."[23]

More recently the real concern over the possibility of transfusing the HIV virus into open-heart surgery patients in bank blood has brought about renewed interest in the technique and widespread usage has come about.

The hazards of autotransfusion, primarily air embolism, still exist, though improvements in equipment have gone far to minimize this danger.[24] Safety devices on current automated equipment help guard against this possibility. To be effective, however, the user must utilize the safety features in the manner in which the manufacturer designed and advised their use. Not to turn on alarms, or to circumvent the safety features, places the patient in jeopardy.

Disseminated intravascular coagulation (DIC) has largely been avoided due to better anticoagulation as well as cell washing of the salvaged blood. During washing, the thrombin-like substances which are produced by the mechanical and chemical trauma of suctioning and blood cell recovery are removed from the perfusate, and thus DIC is not initiated.

Blood from any operative sight or wound may be salvaged, particularly during a life-threatening emergency. Autotransfusion has and is being utilized for hip replacements, laminectomies, repair of thoracic and abdominal aneurysms, gunshot and knife wounds of the chest and abdomen, to mention only a few applications.

Although the new automated systems are more convenient, any sterile suction system, collecting reservoir, and filtration system may be used. The heart-lung machine and its customary disposable equipment are the logical choice as a readily available system. Suction should be controlled as in any open-heart case (see Chapter 13: CONDUCT OF PERFUSION). A filtered reservoir should not be used in this circumstance due to the

EXPERIMENTS

ON THE

TRANSFUSION OF BLOOD

BY THE

SYRINGE.

BY JAMES BLUNDELL, M.D.

LECTURER ON PHYSIOLOGY AT GUY'S HOSPITAL.

COMMUNICATED

BY MR. CLINE.

Read Feb. 3, 1818.

A FEW months ago I was requested to visit a woman who was sinking under uterine hemorrhagy. The discharge had stopped before my arrival, but her fate was decided, and notwithstanding every exertion of the medical attendants, she died in the course of two hours.

Reflecting afterwards on this melancholy scene, for there were circumstances which gave it a peculiar interest, I could not forbear considering, that the patient might very probably have been saved by transfusion; and that, although there was little

Figure 21.1 Title page from Blundell's first publication on autotransfusion.

A

PRACTICAL TREATISE

ON

PARTURITION,

COMPRISING THE

ATTENDANT CIRCUMSTANCES AND DISEASES OF THE PREGNANT AND PUERPERAL STATES.

BY SAMUEL ASHWELL,

MEMBER OF THE ROYAL COLLEGE OF SURGEONS, AND OF THE MEDICO-CHIRURGICAL SOCIETY OF LONDON.

TO WHICH ARE APPENDED,

TWO PAPERS,

THE ONE CONTAINING SOME REMARKS ON ABDOMINAL SURGERY, THE OTHER ON TRANSFUSION;

PRESENTED BY DR. BLUNDELL,

OF GUY'S HOSPITAL.

SEQUERE NATURAM

LONDON:

PRINTED FOR THOMAS TEGG, 73, CHEAPSIDE;

S. HIGHLEY, FLEET STREET; J. LECKIE, DUBLIN; BELL & BRADFUTE, EDINBURGH; AND R. GRIFFIN & CO. GLASGOW.

1828.

Figure 21.2 Title page from Blundell's second publication on autotransfusion.

extremely high probability of clot formation due to lack of proper heparinization. Salvaged blood is more easily transferred from a clotted non-filtered reservoir than from one which has an integral filter.

External cardiotomy filtration is a must in this situation. The filter will probably be the first part of the system that exhibits clot formation and is the easiest part to change. While changing a cardiotomy filter, blood salvage can continue uninterrupted, thus providing the operating surgeon with a relatively clear operative field.

Two suctions should be available with independent suction sources (two different pumpheads or two different wall suction sources). A roller pump should be used to reinfuse the salvaged fluid, or alternatively, the blood should be transferred to blood bags and reinfused through IV or CVP lines using blood infusion pressure devices and proper filtration, the choice, of course, being that of the anesthesiologist (see Figure 21.3). **The salvage reservoir must not be pressurized** as a pressure infusion system or to increase the speed of transfusion. To do so carries the risk of air embolism or rupture of the system.

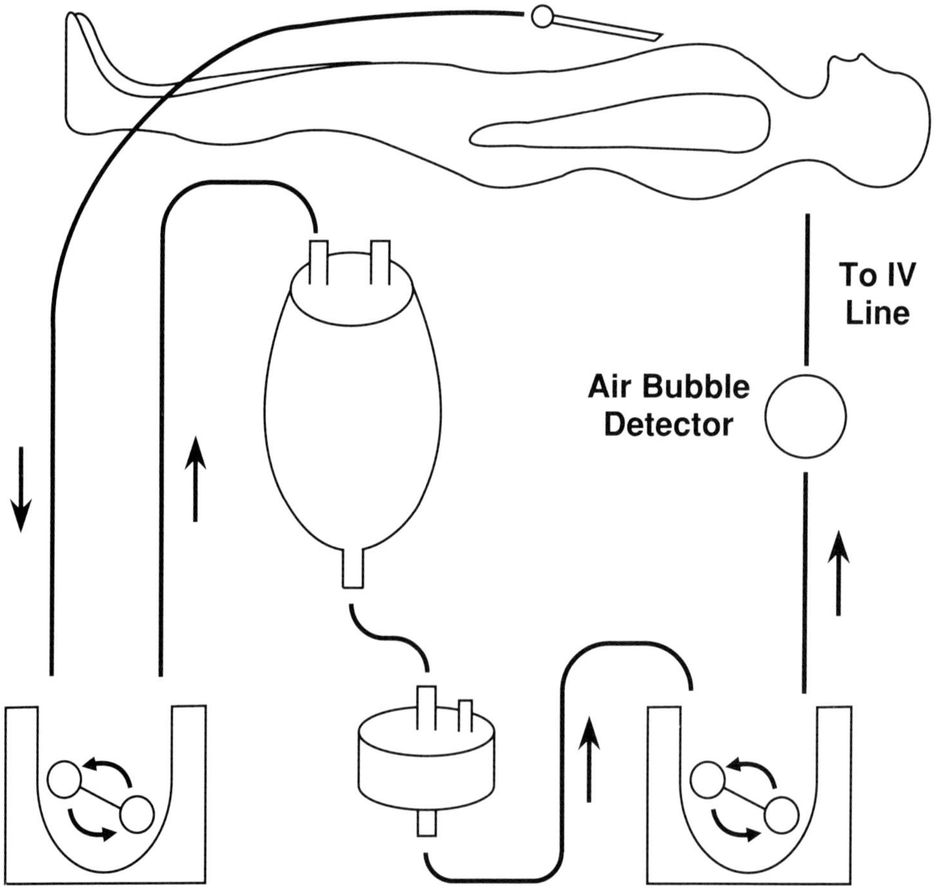

Figure 21.3 Diagram of a typical autotransfusion set-up using readily available roller pumps and cardiotomy reservoir. Note that fluid return to the patient is by positive control roller pump with an inline air bubble detector.

During operation of the suction system various techniques have been tried to avoid clot formation. Dipping the sucker in a heparinized lactated Ringer's solution or normal saline solution intermittently has been tried as well as adding anticoagulant directly to the salvage reservoir. One technique of pretreating the reservoir with a 5% albumin solution has also been reported.[25] To date no satisfactory method has been devised. During a hypovolemic emergency, the team simply does not have time or personnel to indulge in these methods of clot formation avoidance.

In a life or death situation the salvaged fluid may be infused directly back to the patient and the consequences, if any, managed postoperatively as best they can be. This is, of course, a medical decision. After all, if hypovolemia was the cause of death and salvaged fluid was not reinfused because it was contaminated or had not been washed properly, then improper use of the technique may well have been the proximate cause of death. The only limitation in this situation would be that the salvaged fluid must be passed through a proper filter on its way into the patient. These authors recommend use of a cardiotomy filter of the combined depth and screen type. The infusion rate in this circumstance will be dictated by both the availability of salvaged fluid and the needs of the patient.

The hazard of infusion of an air embolus in these circumstances is increased dramatically. The emergent needs of the moment, a higher emotional intensity in the operating room setting, an increase in the volume and noise level of conversation, as well as the number of interrupted and overlapping conversations all will contribute to the possibility of

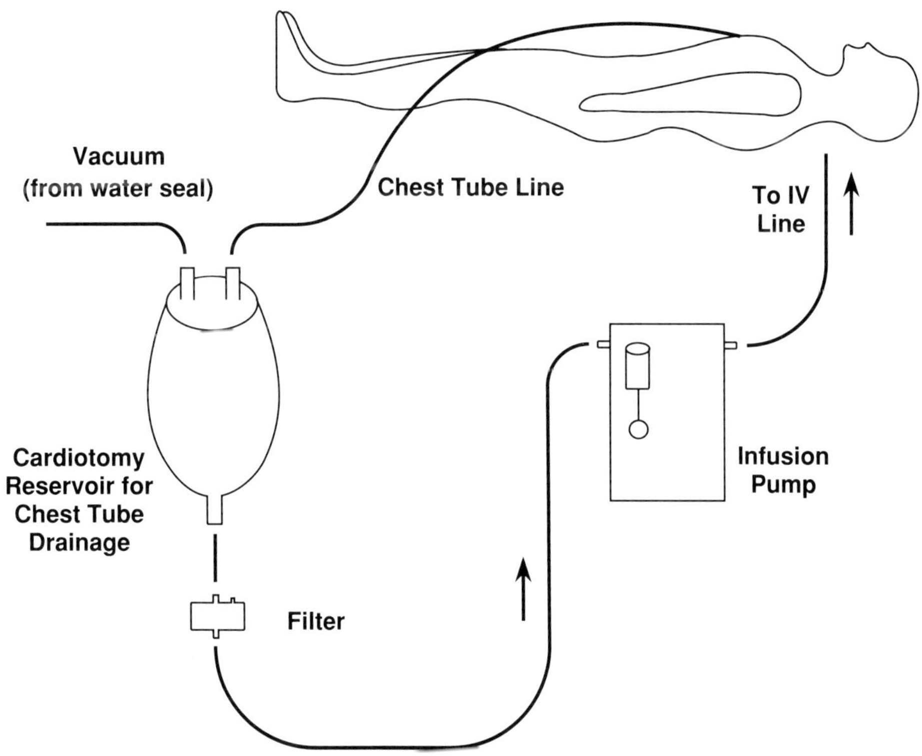

Figure 21.4 Diagram of cardiotomy reservoir, previously used on patient for cardiopulmonary bypass surgery, utilized on same patient for Recovery/ICU chest tube drainage recovery and autotransfusion by IMED type infusion pump. The infusion pump should have automatic air detector shut off alarm. Extracorporeal filter may be changed if clotting occurs.

a mistake on the part of the autotransfusion operator. Placed in this setting, the operator must be at their highest level of concentration and awareness.

Time permitting, the salvaged fluid may be properly processed by the Blood Bank. Almost all hospital Blood Banks today have the capability of cell washing for processing frozen blood. The Blood Bank can concentrate the red blood cells and then properly wash the packed red cells before sending them back to the operating room for transfusion into the patient. This is the preferable technique. Commercial systems are readily available which will accomplish all of this in the operating room and will do it inline.

The techniques described above are for those settings and institutions who have chosen not to spend the thousands of dollars for the permanent equipment. The automated systems are self explanatory, however, the danger is ever-present of air embolism regardless of the system employed. These authors believe that it is a misutilization of personnel to have cardiopulmonary perfusionists operate cell salvaging equipment as a primary responsibility.

The most useful application of autotransfusion in which the perfusionist is involved is the utilization of the technique of mediastinal or chest drainage autotransfusion following cardiopulmonary bypass.[26] This is a valuable and inexpensive method of avoiding postoperative transfusion in the Recovery/ICU period unless massive blood loss is encountered.

The cardiotomy reservoir that was used during the cardiopulmonary bypass procedure is connected to the mediastinal/chest drainage tubes on the inlet side of the reservoir. The outlet side of the reservoir is connected to an IV line with an infusion pump inline. All unused reservoir inlets are blocked, usually by using short pieces of tubing to connect the inlets to each other. The remaining inlet is connected to an underwater sealed suction (see Figure 21.4). This regulated constant suction drains shed blood into the cardiotomy reservoir where it may be filtered and returned to the patient. A filtered cardiotomy reservoir is more likely to clot in this application, and is thus another reason to use an unfiltered reservoir and external cardiotomy filtration (see Chapter 8: FILTRATION).

Blood loss is noted on the usual hourly basis and replaced from the reservoir by infusion through the IV line using an IMED or other suitable infusion pump system (see Figure 21.4). These devices have an inline bubble sensor and will prevent infusion of air emboli if used properly.

Experience has demonstrated that, if the reservoir clots, replacement with a new reservoir will not alleviate the problem. The second reservoir will clot before meaningful autotransfusion has occurred. This should indicate a satisfactory status of the patient's coagulation system and probably the absence of significant bleeders. The autotransfusion system is abandoned at this point even if it occurs while the patient is still in the operating room. To persist with autotransfusion under these circumstances will only result in frustration for all involved and jeopardize the acceptance of the technique. If significant mediastinal bleeding occurs in the ICU several hours after bypass, the patient will probably meet the criteria for surgical exploration.

REFERENCES

1. Blundell, J: Experiments on the transfusion of blood. Medico Chir Trans 9:56, 1818.
2. Ashwell S: A practical treatise on paturation. London: Thomas Tegg, 1928.
3. Elmendorf: Ueber wiederinfusion nash punktion eines frischen hamatothorax. Munchen. Med Wschr 64:36, 1917.
4. Highmore W: Overlooked source of blood supply for transfusion in post-partum haemorrhage. Lancet 1:89, 1874.
5. Lockwood CD: Surgical treatment of Banti's disease. Surg Gynecol Obstet 25:188, 1917.
6. Davis LE, Cushing H: Experiences with blood replacement during or after major intracranial operations. Surg Gynecol Obstet 40:310, 1925.

7. Schilling JA, Allen JG: Discussion of a paper by Langston HT, Miles G, Dalessandro W: Further experience with autologous blood transfusions. Ann Surg 158:333, 1967.
8. Pathak UN, Stewart DB: Autotransfusion in ruptured ectopic pregnancy. Lancet 1:961, 1970.
9. Dyer RH: Intra-operative autotransfusion, a preliminary report and a new method. Am J Surg 112:510, 1966.
10. Klebanoff G: Early clinical experience with a disposable unit for the intra-operative salvage and reinfusion of blood loss (intra-operative autotransfusion). Am J Surg 120:718, 1970.
11. Dyer RH, Alexander JT, Brighton CT: Atraumatic aspiration of whole blood for intra-operative transfusion. Am J Surg 123:510, 1972.
12. Symbas PN, Levin JM, Ferrier FL, Sybers RG: A study of autotransfusion from hemothorax. Southern Med J 62:671, 1969.
13. Symbas PN: Autotransfusion from hemothorax: Experimental and clinical studies. J Trauma 12:689, 1972.
14. Noon GP, Solis RT, Natelson EA: A simple method of intraoperative autotransfusion. Surg Gynecol Obstet 143:65, 1976.
15. Thurer RL, Hauer JM: Autotransfusion and blood conservation. Curr Probl Surg 19:98, 1982.
16. Duncan SE, Klebanoff G, Rogers W: Patient experience in intraoperative autotransfusion. Rev Surg 31:121, 1974.
17. Reed CC, Milam JD, Sabawala PB, Wukasch DC, Cooley DA: Autotransfusion: New or used? JECT 5:42, 1973.
18. Stehling LC, Zauder HL, Rogers W: Intraoperative autotransfusion. Anesth 43:337, 1975.
19. Kingsley JR, Valeri CR, Peters H: Citrate anti-coagulation and on-line cell washing in intra-operative autotransfusion in the babboon. Surg Forum 24:258, 1973.
20. Rakower SR, Worth MH: Autotransfusion: Perspective and critical problems. J Trauma 13:573, 1973.
21. Brener BJ, Raines JK, Chesney CM, Colman RW, Darling RC: Intra-operative autotransfusion. Surg Forum 24:255, 1973.
22. Dowling J, Brettschneider L: Autotransfusion, its use in the severly injured patient. First Annual Bentley Autotransfusion Seminar, 1973.
23. Duncan J: On re-infusion of blood in primary and other amputations. Br Med J 1192, 1886.
24. Hazard: Air embolism from autotransfusion units. ECRI Hazard Bulletin, July 11, 1986.
25. Kurusz M, Schneider B, Conti VR: Albumin pretreatment of autotransfusion apparatus. JECT 14:467, 1982.
26. Cosgrove DM, Amiot DM, Meserko JM: An improved technique for autotransfusion of shed mediastinal blood. Ann Thoracic Surg 40:519, 1985.

..LAWSUITS AND ...CASENOTES

... The patient was flown in from Elsewhere General Hospital for "a little bleeding from the inferior aortic arch. A few sponges were packed around the bleeding site and the chest closed." The patient was Air Evaced to another hospital. After opening the chest, the surgeon removed 17 lap sponges and discovered the entire inferior aortic arch had been torn. At the last moment before surgery a simple autotransfusion system had been set up which included a 1500 ml hardshell reservoir, a single sucker, and return line to the patient. The return was to the CVP line and was gravity infusion. The autotransfusion system was overwhelmed immediately, and the perfusionist pressurized the reservoir in an attempt to return blood to the patient. The cardiotomy reservoir exploded, spraying the operating room with blood. The patient was pronounced dead on the table.

... The autotransfusion return was to the internal jugular vein and the system had only one suction pump and no return pump. The perfusionist was returning blood to the patient by pressurizing the autotransfusion reservoir. During the procedure his attention was directed elsewhere, the reservoir was pressurized and emptied, and air was pumped into the patient. The patient died on the operating table. Autopsy revealed a patent foramen ovale. The cause of death was massive cerebral arterial air emboli.

... Autotransfusion was being utilized for a trauma case involving multiple injuries. The system incorporated a safety device in the reservoir which would detect the absence of a blood level by reflective light detection of the two wavelengths of blood. The reservoir was emptied of blood and the patient died of massive air emboli. Upon examination a blood clot was discovered in the reservoir. The clot was located directly across from the safety device sensor and was large enough and close enough to reflect the correct wavelength of light in a high enough intensity for the detector to sense a false reading of a blood level in the reservoir.

... The perfusionist operating the autotransfusion system was using pressurization of the reservoir to return blood to the patient. The reservoir emptied and air emboli were transfused into the patient. The patient died, the patient suffered no ill effect, the patient suffered neurological problems postoperatively. NOTE: This accident has been reported repeatedly. The authors estimate between 25 and 55 accidents of this nature have occurred and been reported and perhaps twice that number have gone unreported.

... An automated autotransfusion system incorporating an inline cell washer was being used in the manual mode. The system was allowed to run dry and the reinfusion bag was directly connected to the patient. Air was pumped into the patient at a rate of 5 ml per second for an indeterminate length of time. The patient died of massive air emboli. Operating the system in the manual mode disengaged the safety alarms integral to the system. NOTE: The same accident with the same results occurred at separate hospitals two weeks apart.

... In a single pump autotransfusion set-up, an extracorporeal screen filter was placed between the collection reservoir and the distal IV tubing. The roller pump was used to simultaneously suction blood from the operative site and to pressurize the reservoir. In an attempt to return all the salvaged blood to the patient, the perfusionist pressurized the reservoir to force blood through a screen filter. About the same time, the anesthesiologist heard a loud gurgling noise through an esophageal stethoscope. The filter was noted to be one-third full, but the IV line between the filter and patient was filled with air. A sternotomy was rapidly performed, and 200 ml of air was evacuated from the right atrium. The patient was successfully resuscitated, recovered, and was discharged from the hospital with no ill effects.

Chapter 22:

CIRCULATORY SUPPORT AND IABP

Chapter 22: CIRCULATORY SUPPORT AND IABP

The intra-aortic balloon pump (IABP) has been widely used for temporary cardiac assist for two decades,[1] and virtually all open-heart programs have an IABP available. While the IABP may be used in medical or surgical patients, failure to wean the patient from cardiopulmonary bypass is a primary application.[2] The Survey revealed an estimated overall usage of IABP for this problem at 3%. Additionally, cardiac, or circulatory assist devices other than the IABP, had been used by 41% of the respondents in 450 cases during the 36-month study period, 1982 to 1985. While the role of perfusionists during circulatory support using these devices is evolving at the present, like ECMO, it is likely that perfusionists will become involved or exposed at some point to circulatory support devices other than conventional cardiopulmonary bypass.

INTRA-AORTIC BALLOON PUMP

Techniques used to facilitate safe intra-aortic balloon pumping during cardiopulmonary bypass include, first and foremost, a second perfusionist or qualified person to operate the IABP. It is lethal for a perfusionist to operate a heart-lung machine and an IABP at the same time. While perfusionists are sometimes forced into this situation with no patient injury resulting, there have been other cases when the perfusionist was so preoccupied with operation of the IABP, that a massive air embolism accident occurred from the cardiopulmonary bypass circuit and the patient died. Therefore, the authors consider it **mandatory that a perfusionist never operate a heart-lung machine and an IABP simultaneously.**

Because the need for IABP during cardiac surgery is unpredictable, it is prudent to have a designated ECG cable available for IABP triggering. This can be accomplished by using an approach that utilizes "pre problem planning" on all open-heart patients. The time saved and activity minimized if an IABP is needed can make the implementation to IABP assistance during cardiopulmonary bypass smooth. The ECG signal can be "slaved" to the IABP from the routine ECG monitor during surgery, and more permanent leads may be applied postoperatively before transporting the patient to ICU/recovery.

Having a good ECG signal is crucial to reliable IABP triggering and accurate timing. Use of an electrocautery suppression insert in the cable can also provide a reliable ECG trigger when electrocautery is being used. Alternatively, most IABPs can be triggered by the arterial pressure waveform if it is of sufficient amplitude. Disadvantages may include double triggering when the IABP inflation wave form occurs and loss of trigger when the arterial line transducer is turned off for blood sampling. Alternatively, a pulmonary artery pacing catheter may be used as a source of an intraventricular ECG.[3] This signal is reportedly not affected by surgical electrocautery. Conventional skin surface leads, however, are placed after the patient is undraped or in the ICU.

A recently recognized risk with IABP during cardiopulmonary bypass is massive air embolism if IABP deflation should occur when the aorta is opened, for example during insertion or removal of either the aortic or cardioplegia cannula. The sudden vacuum created by balloon deflation can draw a large quantity of room air into the aorta with fatal consequences. Therefore, the IABP should be turned off whenever the surgeon opens the aorta. Obviously, close communication is required between the surgeon and IABP operator to avoid this complication.

The issue of whether to inflate the IABP while on bypass is not clear, and this usually is a medical decision that varies depending on institutional protocol. Of course, during the period of cardioplegia with no QRS complex, the IABP cannot be triggered by the patient's

ECG. Intra-aortic balloon pump manufacturers recommend that the IABP be inflated periodically by using the built-in trigger. The rate is adjustable and the frequency of pumping can be reduced to 1:3, 1:4 or 1:8. The rationale for intermittently inflating the IABP while on bypass is to decrease the risk of thrombus developing on the static IABP which still may occur even in a fully heparinized patient. The IABP should never be permitted to remain deflated for more than 45 to 60 minutes.

A purported advantage of inflating the IABP more frequently during cardiopulmonary bypass is that it provides "pulsatile perfusion." This may persuade everyone that the patient is being better perfused because it may look more physiologic, but the authors believe it has little proven value (see Chapter 9: BLOOD PUMPS AND PULSATILE FLOW).

When an IABP is being used and the patient is having open-heart surgery, the IABP console must be carefully positioned in the operating room so that it will not interfere with the bypass lines, oxygenator, reservoirs, etc. or with the perfusionist who is operating the heart-lung machine. Using IABP catheter extension tubing permits more flexibility in avoiding crowded conditions near the heart-lung machine. The IABP console should be plugged into a different wall outlet than that one used for the heart-lung machine and preferably one on a separate circuit to avoid electrical overload with possible loss of power during cardiopulmonary bypass.

When an IABP is in place and used for weaning the patient from bypass, no special techniques are used. However, several attempts may be required as the anesthesiologist adjusts drug dosages to obtain optimum cardiac ejection. Weaning may be prolonged and the perfusionist must avoid overfilling the heart which often occurs more quickly in patients with a poorly beating ventricle. Close coordination and essential communication among surgeon, perfusionist and anesthesiologist are required under this trying circumstance (see Chapter 3: INTERFACE).

CENTRIFUGAL PUMP

Despite the success of IABP in weaning patients from bypass, other, more effective ventricular assist devices (VADs) are sometimes used. The centrifugal pump was initially designed to function as an artificial heart, but it has seen increasing use as the arterial pump during bypass. Since 1980, it has also been used as a VAD for prolonged periods, and in some centers it has been used as a "bridge" to cardiac transplantation.

The popularity of the centrifugal pump was evident from The Survey data. Of 450 cardiac assist cases (excluding IABP) the centrifugal pump was used 54% of the time. The reasons for this probably relate to its simplicity and widespread availability and the misconception that less heparin could be used during support procedures.

The centrifugal pump VAD circuit is assembled using conventional thick-walled polyvinyl chloride (PVC) tubing in a preassembled sterile pack including the pumphead and other components. The section of the circuit containing the pumphead is passed from the sterile field leaving enough length of inlet and outlet tubing on the table to reach the patient's heart. The centrifugal pumphead is positioned on the console with the outlet facing downward to retard air embolism if any enters the circuit.

Priming the centrifugal pump can be accomplished by either syringe filling or applying vacuum to either the inlet or outlet tubing while immersing the other end in a basin of saline or balanced electrolyte solution. Once filled, the centrifugal pump should be briefly recirculated to thoroughly displace any residual air. Positioning the outlet facing upward can facilitate priming and deairing. The design of current centrifugal pumps eliminates the need for carbon dioxide flushing. Some type of flow meter is required with a centrifugal pump because flow is pressure dependent; i.e., the flow will vary at a given RPM depending upon resistance at the outlet side or in the patient. The flow meter may be either inline or a clamp-on type, and the electronics for displaying blood flow are built into current centrifugal pump consoles. An accessory Y should be placed on the pump outflow side for pressure measurement or a blood access site.

Cannulation for left VAD placement typically is from the left atrium to aorta. Most surgeons use the same aortic cannulation site and cannula that was used for bypass. A 28 to 32 Fr wire-wound venous cannula is used for the left atrial cannulation. Left ventricular cannulation has been shown experimentally to decompress the left ventricle and decrease myocardial oxygen consumption more effectively,[3-6] however the left atrial site is used most frequently clinically to avoid damage to the apex of the poorly functioning left ventricle. Some surgeons may advance the left atrial cannula through the mitral valve and into the left ventricle. From a technical standpoint, however, operation of the LVAD is no different with either approach (see Figure 22.1).

A gravity-fed reservoir should be interposed between the heart and the centrifugal pump. Even a centrifugal pump can create enough negative pressure to aspirate air in around the left atrial cannula if the purse-string sutures are not totally sealed. Gravity drainage is the safest method to supply blood to the centrifugal pump. With a reservoir in the drainage line to the pump, unloading of the left heart is more easily controlled without the necessity of increasing the arterial return to the patient.

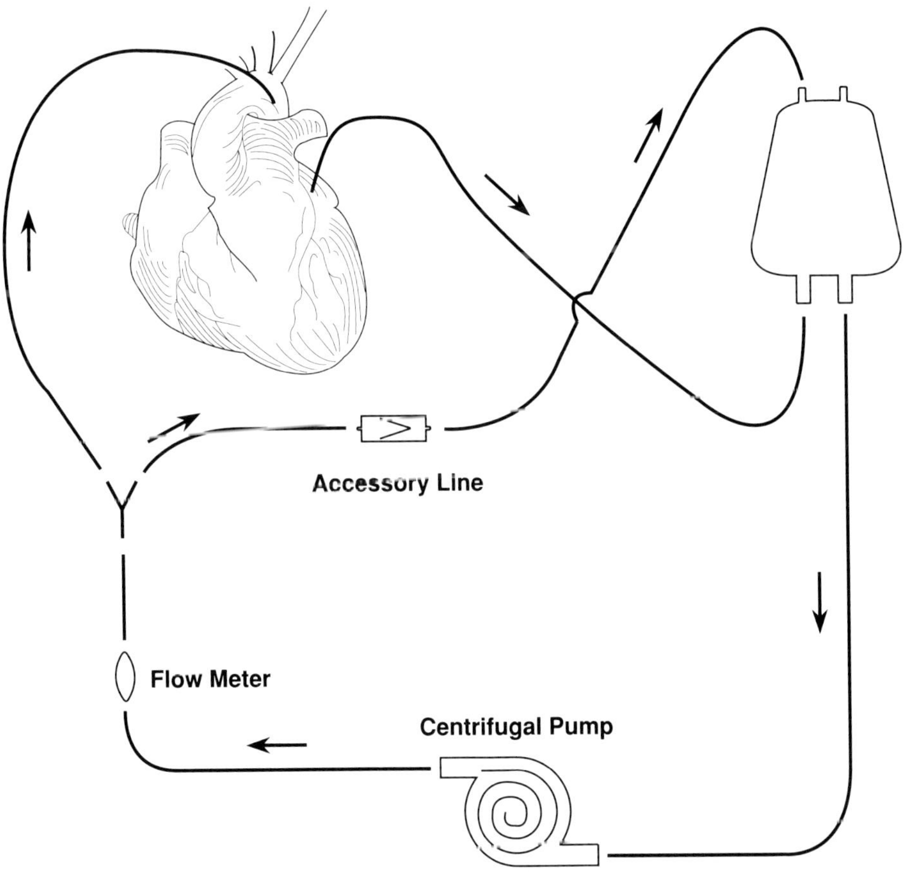

Figure 22.1 LVAD set-up with reservoir and centrifugal pump. Note accessory line Y distal to the pumphead and flowmeter.

Because of the risk of arterial embolization (particulate or air) some have advocated that aortic cannulation be in the descending thoracic aorta just distal to the left subclavian artery.[7] This practice makes sense to these authors, but it is a surgical decision. Alternatively, screen arterial filters have been used during long-term circulatory support,[8] but this practice appears to be not widely used with VADs.

When a centrifugal pump is used to wean a patient from bypass, and after the left atrial cannula has been placed and connected to the primed pump, the arterial flow is slowly decreased until the left atrial pressure (LAP) and/or pulmonary wedge pressure (PWP) rises to 15 to 20 mmHg. Bypass is stopped and the centrifugal pump outflow line is connected to the previously used aortic cannula. The same deairing procedures are used when making a conventional extracorporeal tubing connection. The centrifugal pump is then turned on and the flow is increased until the LAP or PWP begins to fall. The flow in the centrifugal pump is generally set to a cardiac index of 2.2 to 2.5 L/min/m^2, but higher flows are sometimes required. The LAP or PWP must remain greater than 5 to 10 mmHg by adding volume to the patient or regulating flow from the pump.

Despite the fact that a centrifugal pump is not considered a positive displacement type as is the roller pump, some negative pressure is exerted on the pump inlet side, and air can be aspirated into the pump where it may remain trapped, or it can embolize to the patient's systemic circulation (see Chapter 25: AIR).

Patients with an LVAD usually will have an IABP placed initially, and the technical considerations are the same as previously discussed with the exception that another piece of equipment requiring extra personnel will be crowding the already busy operating room. The perfusionist in this situation must not become distracted from operating the heart-lung machine. It must be remembered that these patients at this stage are usually normothermic and at full cardiopulmonary flow so there is less margin for error.

If the patient exhibits a low LAP or PWP with LVAD support, and the central venous pressure (CVP) is high (>20 to 25 mmHg), right ventricular failure may be present. Under these circumstances the medical decision may be made to support the right ventricle if varying the pharmacological therapy does not improve patient hemodynamics. An IABP placed in the pulmonary artery (IPABP) has been used,[9-12] most likely out of desperation, and some patients have survived with conventional IABP and an IPABP. However, The Survey revealed, out of 192 such cases, a patient outcome of 80% mortality.

A balloon placed in the pulmonary artery can reduce the afterload of the failing right ventricle and assist pulmonary blood flow, but obviously does nothing for coronary perfusion. Timing the IPABP therefore should be aimed at maximum augmentation and endiastolic unloading as assessed by the pulmonary artery pressure waveform.[13]

A more effective and accepted method of right ventricular assist is use of an RVAD. Like LVAD, an RVAD may be either a roller pump or centrifugal type, with the centrifugal used most often. Cannulation is via the right atrium and pulmonary artery. If a single right atrial cannula has been used for bypass, it may be used for RVAD (see Figure 22.2).

If LVAD and RVAD pumps are used the flows from each pump must be carefully coordinated to avoid inducing pulmonary edema in the patient. Because each ventricle may be marginally functioning and contributing some output, coordination is assessed by the LAP and CVP. Flows from both pumps therefore may not be equal.

The LAP is lowered to approximately 5 mmHg by slowly increasing the LVAD flow, and the RVAD flow is then slowly increased until the LAP rises to approximately 15 mmHg. The LVAD/RVAD flows are increased stepwise in this manner until the LVAD flow is at a cardiac index of 2.2 to 2.5 L/min/m^2. Any changes in either pump flow should be done slowly and must be assessed by observing the effects on filling pressures. Numerous adjustments are often required, and if the LVAD flow cannot be increased up to 2.2

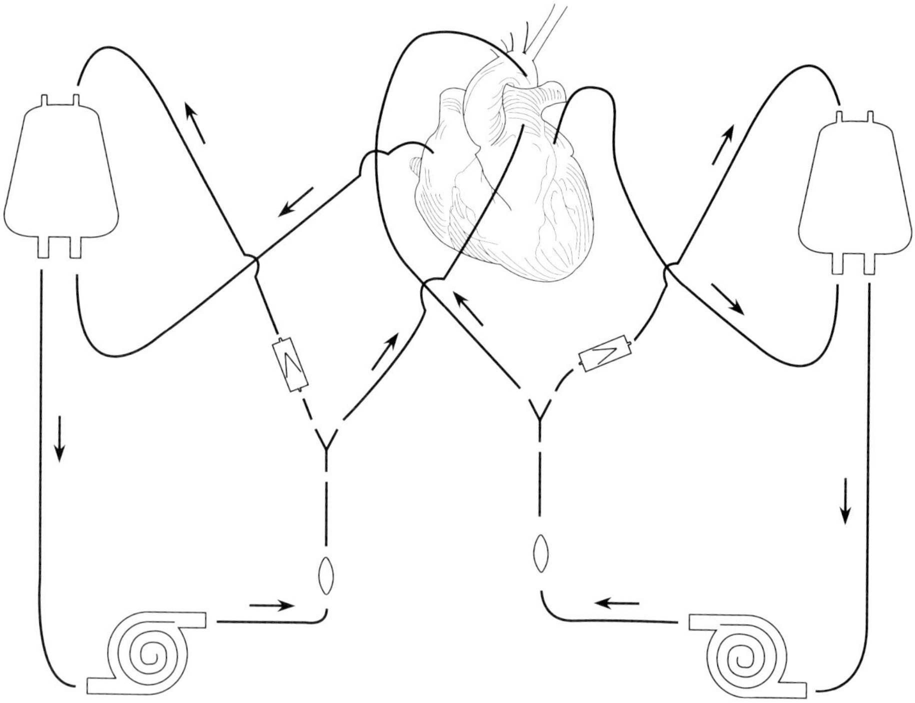

Figure 22.2 LVAD-RVAD set-up.

L/min/m^2, fluid additions are required. Other reasons for not being able to achieve 2.2 L/min/m^2 during biventricular assist are cannula malpositioning or clot formation, both of which may be difficult to determine.

Anticoagulation was initially not thought necessary with a centrifugal pump,[13] but most teams maintain the activated clotting time (ACT) between 150 to 250 seconds during circulatory assist with a centrifugal pump. Because thrombus formation is highly dependent on flow conditions, it is essential that the ACT be maintained greater than 200 seconds if the pump flow is less than 1 L/min as occurs during weaning.

Transportation of a patient from the operating room to ICU who has an IABP, LVAD and/or RVAD connected is a challenge. Enough personnel must be available to assist during transport to allow the devices to be safely managed and monitored. Kinking or stretching vital lines is always a risk. The VAD(s) and IABP(s) should be equipped with battery power and pneumatic sources if continuous circulatory assistance is to be maintained during the transfer. In the absence of battery power, or in the event the battery is dead, a handcrank drive may be used. Alternatively, two long electrical extension cords can be used as the patient is wheeled from outlet to outlet.

Placement of a small (300 to 500cc) flexible reservoir bag in the LVAD or RVAD inlet line will offer the advantage of additional assessment of volume status independent of patient filling pressures. Such a reservoir also has the added advantage of a blood return site if an ultrafiltration device is used. Presence of a reservoir bag in the RVAD circuit also facilitates the addition of a membrane oxygenator if ECMO is needed for pulmonary failure.

Myocardial recovery and weaning the patient from circulatory assist rarely occurs earlier than 24 to 36 hours of cardiac support, but apparently if hemodynamic improvement does not occur within 72 hours it is unlikely to occur at all. It is accomplished by slowly decreasing the VAD flow which will cause the filling pressures (LAP and/or CVP) to rise. At 15 to 20 mmHg, strong ventricular ejections should be seen if the ventricles are recovering. The weaning process may be prolonged over several hours, and further reductions in VAD flow are determined by measuring cardiac outputs, assessing clinical signs, and on-going medical management. The primary technique consideration during the weaning is to maintain adequate anticoagulation by frequent ACT measurements.

The criteria for electively changing out the centrifugal pumphead is not established. The manufacturers recommend that it be performed every 24 hours. However, clinical cases have been done with one pumphead used continuously for more than a week. The concern is clot or thrombus formation in the device at areas of low flow. Such thrombi can embolize with deleterious consequences for the patient (e.g., stroke or peripheral ischemia).

One technique to assess thrombus formation is to briefly come off assist by stopping flow and clamping the outflow line. The pumphead is removed from the console and inspected with the aid of a flashlight to determine if clots have formed near the center of the centrifugal pump. If the decision is made to change pumpheads, the inlet and outlet tubing are double clamped near the pumphead, sterilized, and transected with a sterile scapel blade or scissors. The inlet tubing from the patient is connected to the inlet side of the new pumphead and the inlet clamp is slowly released to fill the pumphead and expel air. Gentle tapping and rotating will facilitate this procedure. All air is excluded when the outlet tubing is connected to the outlet of the pumphead. After this is accomplished the new pumphead is inserted in the console and flow is reestablished. The entire pumphead changeout can be accomplished expeditiously in less than 45 seconds. The primary technique considerations are to avoid air, minimize blood loss, and maintain sterility when the new connections are being made.

Slight hypothermia may occur in the patient receiving centrifugal circulatory assist. This has not been a significant problem, but one group[15] has suggested wrapping a topical cooling device around the pumphead and recirculating water from a warming blanket heater to prevent hypothermia which may exacerbate cardiac arrhythmias. Patient hypothermia can also be prevented with warming blankets or overhead radiant warmer.

ROLLER PUMP

While technically less acceptable, a conventional roller pump may be used for prolonged circulatory assistance. It was the second most commonly used assist pump (30% of 450 cases) in The Survey. Disadvantages include, first, the risk of air aspiration from the outflow cannulation site if filling pressures fall below 5 mmHg, and secondly, pumphead tubing wear which is manifested by spallation or outright rupture.

If a roller pump is used, a reservoir and arterial filter should be incorporated into the circuit on the pump inflow and outflow lines, respectively. Because pressures must be carefully and continuously monitored, some sort of servo-regulation is advisable to control the roller pump. Additionally, the pumphead tubing segment must be replaced every 24 hours if standard PVC is used. Some have found that lightly lubricating the rollers and tubing with mineral oil will decrease wear and prolong its use. Use of new tubing types (e.g., Tygon S-65-HL) is recommended (see Chapter 23: ECMO). Because of the disadvantages outlined above, however, the authors do not recommend that a roller pump be used for prolonged circulatory assist.

ARTIFICIAL HEART

Sac-type, pneumatic or electrically powered ventricular pumps with prosthetic valves are increasingly being used as a "bridge" to cardiac transplantation. The role of perfusionists with this technology is currently unresolved, and the few centers that implant these devices in patients generally have a designated circulatory support team to manage the devices. While perfusionists may become involved in operating the artificial heart,[16] this practice should be viewed as optional, voluntary, and outside the duties and responsibilities of the perfusionist in these authors' opinion (see Chapter 1: DUTIES AND RESPONSIBILITIES).

Technique considerations during cardiopulmonary bypass for cardiac transplantation when an artificial heart is supporting the patient's circulation revolve around the extra equipment and personnel in the operating room as discussed previously. Obviously, close coordination among the teams participating in such an endeavor must be directed by the surgeon-in-charge.

Perhaps the most important technique consideration when prolonged circulatory support is used is to maintain strict aseptic techniques. Like ECMO, VADs are used in the ICU setting which are subject to more nosocomial organisms. Perfusionists who participate in managing VADs should always be concerned with sterility. Reverse isolation techniques can minimize infectious complications whenever prolonged circulatory support devices are used.

REFERENCES

1. Kantrowitz A, Tjonneland S, Freed PS, Phillips SJ, Butner AN, Sherman Jr JL: Initial clinical experience with intra-aortic balloon pumping in cardiogenic shock. JAMA 203:113, 1968.
2. Mundth ED, Yurchak PM, Buckley MJ, Leinbach RC, Kantrowitz A, Austen WG: Circulatory assistance and emergency direct coronary artery surgery for shock complicating acute myocardial infarction. N Eng J Med 283:1382, 1970.
3. Lichtenthal PR, Collins JT: Multipurpose pulmonary artery catheter (Correspondence). Ann Thorac Surg 36:493, 1983.
4. Pierce WS, Aaronson AE, Prophet GA, Williams DR, Waldhausen JA: Hemodynamic and metabolic studies during two types of left ventricular bypass. Surg Forum 23:176, 1972.
5. Laks H, Ott RA, Standeven JW, Hahn JW, Blair OM, Willman VL: The effect of left atrial-to-aortic assistance on infarct size. Circulation 56 (Suppl II):II-38, 1977.
6. Pennock JL, Pae Jr WE, Pierce WS, Waldhausen JA: Reduction of myocardial infarct size: Comparison between left atrial and left ventricular bypass. Circulation 59:275, 1979.
7. Dembitsky WP, Raney AA, Daily PO: Temporary extracorporeal postoperative circulatory support using the roller or rotor impeller pump. Ch. 5 in *Perioperative Cardiac Dysfunction,* Vol 3, Utley JR (Ed), Baltimore: Williams and Wilkins, 1985, pp 63.
8. Peters JL, McRea JC, Fukumasu H, Kolff WJ: Transapical left ventricular bypass (TALVB) without an auxiliary ventricle. Trans Am Soc Artif Intern Org 22:357, 1976.
9. Miller DC, Moreno-Cabral RJ, Stinson EG, Shinn JA, Shumway NE: Pulmonary artery balloon counterpulsation for acute right ventricular failure. J Thorac Cardiovasc Surg 80:760, 1980.
10. Flege Jr JB, Wright CB, Reisinger TJ: Successful balloon counterpulsation for right ventricular failure. Ann Thorac Surg 37:167, 1984.
11. Moran JM, Opravil M, Gorman AJ, Rastegar H, Meyers SN, Michaelis LL: Pulmonary artery balloon counterpulsation for right ventricular failure: II. Clinical experience. Ann Thorac Surg 38:254, 1984.
12. Symbas PN, McKeown PP, Santora AH, Vlasis SE: Pulmonary artery balloon counterpulsation for treatment of intraoperative right ventricular failure. Ann Thorac Surg 39:437, 1985.
13. Opravil M, Gorman AJ, Krejcie TC, Michaellis LL, Moran JM: Pulmonary artery balloon counterpulsation for right ventricular failure: I. Experimental results. Ann Thorac Surg 38:242, 1984.
14. Dixon CM, Magovern GJ: Evaluation of the BioPump for long-term cardiac support without heparinization. JECT 14:331, 1982.
15. Young JN, Belz R, Iverson LIG, Ennix Jr CL, Ecker RR, May RD, Masterson R, May IA: A technique for avoidance of hypothermia during prolonged mechanical circulatory support with centrifugal pumps. Ann Thorac Surg 44:90, 1987.
16. Smith DL, Hastings WL, Joyce LD, DeVries WC: Management of the artifical heart driver; A new role for the perfusionist? JECT 16:18, 1984.

..LAWSUITS AND ...CASENOTES

... A patient was admitted with an acute myocardial infarction followed by cardiac arrest while awaiting operation. After successful resuscitation an IAPB was inserted without incident. Two days later, with improved hemodynamics, the decision was made to remove the balloon. Acetone was used to remove adhesive tape from the skin and from around the catheter. Shortly thereafter the catheter softened and then fractured completely. The catheter stump was clamped and withdrawn without difficulty.

... The IAPB was inserted, but difficulty was encountered in attempting to pass the balloon trans-femorally. The balloon was then inserted through a dacron graft to the ascending aorta. It functioned normally for 34 hours with the leak detector turned off. Blood was noticed in the clear tubing to the balloon console. The pump was shut off. The balloon was removed. The patient suffered no ill effects. Several abraided areas were found on the balloon, one of which had perforated the balloon.

... During cardiopulmonary using a Pulsatile Assist Device (PAD) the PAD ruptured and massive air emboli were pumped into the patient. The patient expired.

... During LVAD with a centrifugal pump, the left atrial cannula became malpositioned. The pump sucked air into the pump which then transferred the air into the patient. The patient expired.

Chapter 23:

ECMO CIRCUITS AND TECHNIQUES

Chapter 23: ECMO CIRCUITS AND TECHNIQUES

The application of prolonged extracorporeal membrane oxygenator (ECMO) support is growing, particularly in neonates who fail to respond to conventional mechanical ventilation and medical therapy. The concomitant growth in the number of prolonged ventricular assist cases in adults following cardiac surgery or for the cardiac and/or lung transplant patient awaiting donor organs also comprises a patient group that may benefit from ECMO. The largest clinical experience, however, is for the newborn respiratory failure, and ECMO programs currently are being established in all parts of the country as well as world-wide. The success rates are quite impressive when one considers that the entry criteria for candidates generally predicts a mortality rate of at least 80% in these patients without ECMO. The most recent survival figures for the ECMO central registry in Ann Arbor, Michigan are 81%.[1]

Based on these facts, it is probable that perfusionists may be asked to become involved in ECMO at some point in their career. In this chapter we outline the most common ECMO circuits and techniques that have been used to date. It must be recognized, however, that ECMO techniques are undergoing modification and refinement, and the ECMO components used five years from now will probably differ in many respects from those used currently. Safety and automation along with improved blood surfaces appear to be the major areas of research directed towards these refinements.

The establishment of an ECMO program involves a vast commitment of resources, personnel, time, and money. It is not practical to throw together an ECMO team from staff perfusionists and any other hospital personnel who might express an interest. Specifically, **perfusionists should not be included in the ECMO team.** The perfusionist's educational process and experience did not include ECMO, or if it did, the experience was only a brief introduction. The day-to-day function of the perfusionist is more dynamic, and it is likely that the typical perfusionist will develop dissatisfaction with ECMO responsibilities. More importantly, the open-heart program is likely to suffer if it is operating at optimum capacity for the number of perfusionists employed. Surgery may have to be delayed due to the unavailability of a perfusionist who is involved with an ECMO. It is also quite likely that the frequency of accidents and incidences with the cardiopulmonary bypass circuit will increase due to the fatigue of the perfusion personnel who are doing double-duty with the ECMO team.

The University of Michigan technique has been the one most widely used because most of the early ECMO teams trained there. Dr. Robert Bartlett and colleagues emphasize that the ECMO team should be assembled from interested hospital personnel who may be spared from other duties without interfering with or detracting from other ongoing programs, such as perfusion.[2]

THE ECMO CIRCUIT

The basic ECMO circuit consists of a simplified bypass set-up which is self-contained on a stainless steel cart that easily can be moved to any area of the hospital. ECMO can be undertaken in any ICU setting or even on a regular patient unit if appropriate monitoring, vacuum, and gas sources are available.

The only oxygenator approved for long term support is the Sci-Med (Kolobow) spiral coil silicone rubber membrane. Such FDA approval was granted only recently and after nearly 1,000 successful ECMO cases had been performed using it. Some groups have used microporous membrane oxygenators for ECMO support, but the unpredictable failure rate of these devices make them a poor choice for prolonged ECMO. Failure of a microporous membrane most often is manifested by decreasing gas exchange secondary to plasma proteins seeping through the pores into the gas phase of the device.

The correct size membrane oxygenator must be chosen depending on patient size. Table 23.1 shows the recommended oxygenator sizes according to patient weight and blood flow rates.

PUMP

Controversy exists over which type of pump to use for ECMO, but the largest experience for neonatal ECMO has been with a roller pump. Those with direct drive motors are preferred over belt-driven types because of the demands of continuous reliable operation for up to 300 hours at a time. The roller pump should be properly maintained and calibrated every three months. The roller occluding mechanism must operate smoothly and precisely due to the demands placed on the tubing. The pump speed control should permit smooth operation at low flows (50 to 100 ml/min) as are encountered during patient weaning.

FLOW CONTROL

A vital component of any ECMO circuit is some means of servo-regulating the roller pump. If the roller pump is not servo-regulated to respond to decreases or interruptions in venous drainage, the tubing leading into the pump will collapse as the rollers continue to rotate. Under these conditions, the excessive negative pressure can pull gas out of solution, creating a high risk for gas embolism (see Chapter 7: TUBING AND CIRCUITS). It is unlikely that anybody monitoring a roller pump for several hours can reliably maintain the necessary attention span required to manually respond and slow down or stop the pump under the conditions of prolonged blood pumping. Therefore, the authors are convinced that ECMO or any other prolonged circulatory support procedure utilizing a roller pump should always incorporate some form of servo-regulation to prevent this complication.

Table 23.1 **RECOMMENDED OXYGENATOR SIZES**

SciMed Model No.	0600-2A	0800-2A	1500-2A	2500-2A	3500-2A	4500-2A
Patient Weight (kg)	<8	<11	12-19	20-70	71-95	>95
Blood Flow Rate (ml/min)	<1000	<1200	1000-1800	1800-4500	4000-5500	5000-6500
Priming Volume (ml)	80	100	175	330	450	540
Maximum Gas Flow (L/min)	1.8	2.4	4.5	7.5	10.5	13.5

Most commonly a "bladder-box" in the venous line is used to provide this servo-regulation. The "bladder-box" assembly consists of a spring-loaded plunger connected to a microswitch. The plunger rests on a small silicone rubber bladder (approximately 50 ml volume). Blood normally distends the bladder and compresses the plunger. If venous drainage is interrupted, the bladder will collapse and the plunger will extend, tripping the microswitch that interrupts electrical power to the roller pump and causing it to stop. An alarm also sounds to alert the ECMO specialist of this condition. Figure 23.1 shows the "bladder-box" located within the typical ECMO circuit.

When venous drainage is reestablished, the bladder expands, compresses the plunger, turns off the microswitch, power is returned to the roller pump, and pumping resumes. Advantages of the "bladder-box" method for servo-regulating the roller pump are its extensive clinical experience and simplicity. Disadvantages include the present high cost of the bladder reservoir and poor flow dynamics through the bladder that tend to promote clot formation. Such clots often are observed at disassembly of the ECMO circuit even in patients who have been apparently adequately anticoagulated and apparently properly managed with ACTs. If a clot were to embolize and enter the patient, injury or death could result. Therefore, if small clots are observed in the bladder reservoir, the reservoir must not be manipulated. As long as flow is maintained and the "bladder-box" continues to function, these clots are watched carefully for signs of enlargement. If this situation occurs on additional patients, the anticoagulation protocol and management should be carefully examined.

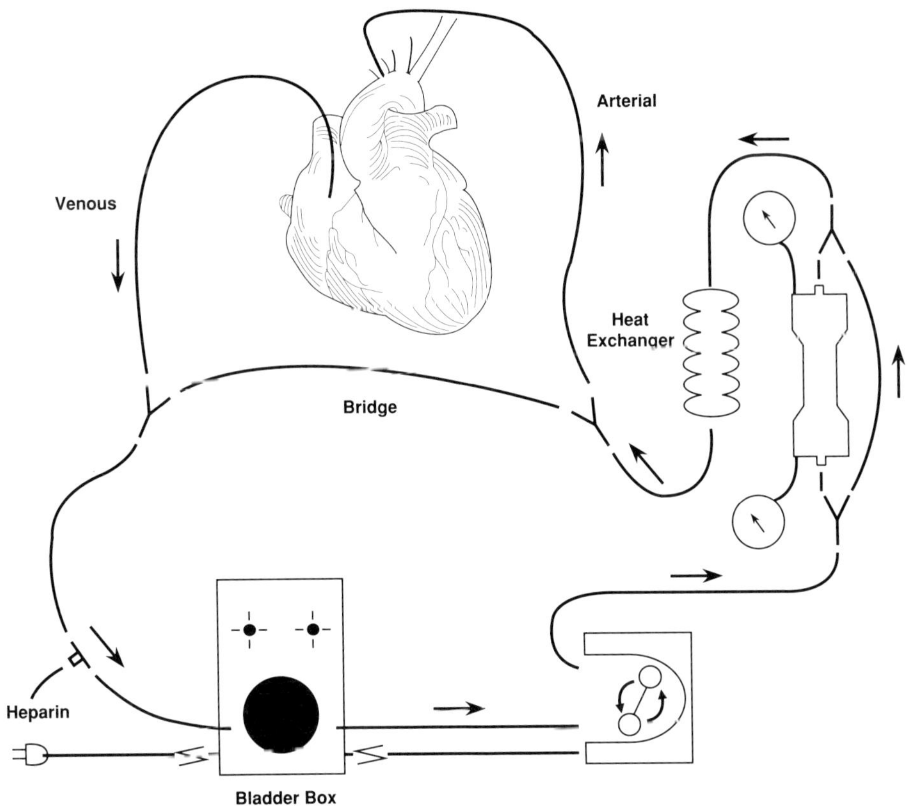

Figure 23.1 Typical neonatal ECMO circuit showing the "bladder box" for servo-regulation of the roller pump.

An alternative technique for flow control is to use pressure transducers before and after the pump. These transducers must be interfaced with a pump control module designed for this purpose. They can be set to slow down or stop the roller pump if either negative pressure is sensed in the line going into the pump or high pressure is sensed in the line coming out of the pump. The advantage of this system is protection against both decreased venous drainage or increased arterial resistance. Both conditions are most often caused by kinked or malpositioned cannulae. Disadvantages of the system are that the transducer controls must be set to the proper limits during set-up, the transducers need to be recalibrated every few hours, and this technique has limited clinical experience.

TUBING

The bypass tubing is PVC which is 1/4" ID with a 3/32" wall thickness. The pumphead section is Tygon S-65-HL tubing which is 1/4" ID with 1/16" wall thickness. If standard PVC tubing is used in the pumphead, an extra contiguous length of tubing is coiled before the pumphead so that worn tubing can be advanced after 24 to 36 hours, or if wear is observed. This is to avoid rupture of tubing and the attendant risks of blood loss, contamination, and air embolism.

Some ECMO teams use polyurethane tubing in the pumphead which is highly resistant to wear. The disadvantage of this tubing is its hardness which can prematurely damage the roller-pump assembly. Other teams use silicone rubber tubing in the roller pumphead, but it is much less resistant to tearing or rupturing in the pumphead and tends to spallate to a greater degree than PVC. It is not recommended for ECMO use by these authors.

TEMPERATURE CONTROL

The patient's temperature is maintained at normothermia by means of an inline heat exchanger. This device also will function as a bubble trap when mounted perpendicular to the floor when blood is pumped into the top and out the bottom. Water supply for the disposable heat exchanger is from a small recirculating water bath as is commonly used for heating pads, although larger units specifically designed for ECMO recently have become available. Some form of inline continuous blood temperature monitoring should be used. Like pediatric patients on total bypass, the body temperature of a neonate can fall more easily than the adult patient.

THE OXYGENATOR

The most common mechanical complication during ECMO is oxygenator failure necessitating replacement. The placement of a membrane bypass line facilitates changing out the oxygenator if it fails due to clotting, inability to oxygenate, or develops leaks. However, the membrane bypass line can be a source of clotting unless it is periodically "flashed" for 3 to 5 seconds. "Flashing" diverts blood flow through the bypass line to clear stagnant blood.

Changing out a membrane during ECMO is facilitated by inclusion of the bypass line, but it carries similar risks to an arterial filter bypass line (see Chapter 8: FILTRATION) One technique to avoid using a bypass line is to place double Y connectors before and after the oxygenator (see Figure 23.2). In this way, a new primed membrane can be added to the circuit without interrupting blood flow to the patient.

Pre and post oxygenator pressures are measured via short extension lines connected to luer-lock ports on the inlet and outlet of the membrane. Knowing the pressure drop, which ranges from 75 to 200 mmHg, permits assessment of membrane function. An increased pressure drop usually signifies development of blood clots in the blood path of the

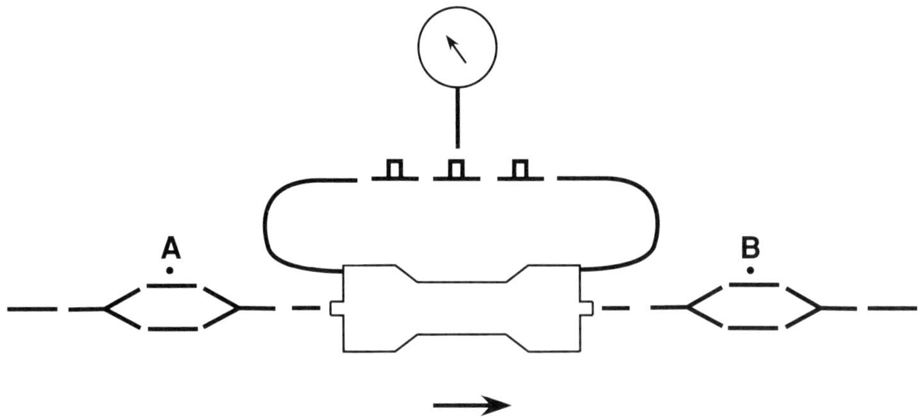

Figure 23.2 Double Y configuration to avoid using a membrane bypass line. Note double clamping at points A and B permits dividing the line and insertion of a newly primed oxygenator in the event that the original oxygenator must be replaced.

oxygenator, although cases of membrane shift have been reported with similar increases in pressure drop.

The decision to change out an oxygenator should be carefully considered and undertaken only when gas exchange is severely compromised. The technique for changing an oxygenator consists of CO_2 flushing, vacuum priming with crystalloid and blood, and carefully inserting the new oxygenator where the bypass line was, or at either end of the double Y connector before and after the oxygenator. Flow through both the original and new oxygenator is briefly alternated until the crystalloid and blood are thoroughly mixed. Once it is confirmed that the new oxygenator is functioning properly, the original one is removed from the circuit.

Gas to the membrane oxygenator during ECMO is supplied from a tank of 95% O_2/5% CO_2 or from an oxygen/air blender. The gas sources may be Y ed together and should include an inline oxygen analyzer to display the percent of oxygen being delivered to the membrane oxygenator and a "pop-off" valve to prevent overpressurization of the gas side. The analyzer and pop-off valve should include an alarm.

Blood gases usually are drawn from an umbilical artery cannula or radial artery line. The percent O_2 saturation can be continuously displayed from a skin probe. Venous O_2 saturation is measured by placing a sensor in the venous return line. Pre and post membrane samples are drawn intermittently to assess gas exchange by the oxygenator.

THE PATIENT

Maintenance fluids, hyperalimentation fluids, and continuous infusion drugs should be administered into the patient as if the patient was not on ECMO. The ECMO circuit can be compromised by infusion of such solutions directly into the circuit with the exception of heparin.

Cannulation for neonatal ECMO is most commonly veno-arterial using the right internal jugular vein and the right common carotid artery. Sometimes the femoral vein is used for venous access.

OPERATION OF THE ECMO CIRCUIT

The ECMO circuit is assembled and primed using aseptic techniques and the oxygenator is CO_2 flushed and has vacuum applied to the gas inlet and outlet to facilitate crystalloid priming and debubbling. Priming the ECMO circuit may differ from institution to institution. It is important that the technique be written in protocol form as several different individuals within an institution may be responsible for priming the circuit on any given case. There also may be long periods between ECMO cases, so having a written protocol will ensure that important details are not omitted.

Heparin administration and the degree of anticoagulation during ECMO are controlled by frequent ACT measurements. Several automated devices are currently used, but because blood loss should be kept to a minimum, a coagulation monitor that requires only 0.2 ml per sample should be chosen.

Blood gases are regulated so that the patient's arterial pO_2 is in the 60 to 80 mmHg range and the pCO_2 is between 35 and 45 mmHg. The patient's lungs may contribute some to the arterial gas partial pressures because ECMO is really partial bypass. An exception is if the heart is completely unloaded and there is only a minimal arterial pulse pressure. If ECMO is used for circulatory support only, the gas exchange requirements from the circuit will be reduced. Oxygen saturations range from 60 to 80% venous and >95% arterial. Typical flow rates are 100 to 150 ml/kg depending on venous and arterial O_2 saturations, arterial pO_2 and clinical signs.

Gowns, gloves, goggles, and masks must be worn around the ECMO patient and procedure. Because of the frequent requirement of blood component transfusion, the possibility of a line coming loose, the possibility of a membrane rupturing, the possibility of exposure to the HIV virus is present, and personnel involved with the ECMO patient must be protected against the risks of blood exposure (see Chapter 6: BLOOD AND BLOOD HANDLING).

Since the procedure will be prolonged and because personnel traffic is heavier than that found in an operating room, strict attention to aseptic technique must be observed. Infusion lines are changed every 24 hours, unused stopcocks ports are kept capped, and the cannulation site dressing is changed daily. Stopcocks should be changed as necessary. Infusion sites are only used for infusion and withdrawal sites are only used for withdrawal.

The hematocrit is maintained at 40 to 45%. If fluid is required due to hypovolemia, fresh frozen plasma or 5% albumin is given if the hematocrit is at or above 45% and packed red blood cells are given if it is lower. Serum calcium levels are monitored and calcium gluconate is given with priming blood or if large volumes of bank blood are given.

Weaning the patient from ECMO is similar to weaning the patient from conventional cardiopulmonary bypass except that it takes several hours. During this time, the mechanical ventilator is turned up to moderate-to-high settings. During trials off ECMO support it is important that the 95% O_2/5% CO_2 tank be turned off and the gas from the blender be turned down, but not off, while recirculating, to avoid excessively high pO_2s while recirculating.

COMPLICATIONS

The most common patient complications associated with ECMO include hemorrhage, neurologic abnormalities, renal insufficiency, and metabolic abnormalities. Mechanical complications occur much less frequently and usually involve oxygenator failure, tubing rupture, pump failure, heat exchanger malfunction, or cannula problems.

Oxygenator failure can sometimes be caused by the accumulation of water vapor condensate in the gas phase. Briefly increasing the gas sweep will clear this water. Tubing rupture has been virtually eliminated with the newer PVC tubing (S-65-HL). Pump failure may be manifested by loss of occlusion or electrical failure. If loss of occlusion occurs,

ECMO must be discontinued while the occlusion is reset. Battery backup for the ECMO cart is advisable as is the availability of a spare roller pump should the primary one malfunction due to internal component failure. Heat exchanger malfunctions (loss of heating or overheating) can be detected by inline temperature probe monitoring and routine observations of patient temperature. Cannula problems most often occur when the baby moves or is lifted for daily weight measurements.

The ECMO specialists must be particularly alert anytime the position of the baby changes. Securing the ECMO venous and arterial lines and absolutely prohibiting personnel between the ECMO cart and the baby will avoid most cannula problems.

In summary, ECMO can be safely undertaken if adequate institutional resources are committed to the program. ECMO specialists must be thoroughly trained in both routine and emergency procedures, and medical management must be clearly established.

REFERENCES

1. Toomasian JM, Snedecor SM, Cornell RE, Cilley RE, Bartlett RH: National experience with extracorporeal membrane oxygenation for newborn respiratory failure; Data from 715 cases. ASAIO Trans 34: 140, 1988.
2. Chapman RA, Toomasian JM, Bartlett RH: *ECMO Specialist Training Manual*, 9th Edition, Ann Arbor, Michigan, Univeristy of Michigan, Extracorporeal Circulation Laboratory and Department of Surgery, 1988.

.. LAWSUITS AND ... CASENOTES

... At autopsy the pathologist found metalic particles in microscopic sections of tissue samples of several ECMO patients who had not survived the procedure. Further investigation revealed that the particles were composed of aluminum. Still further investigation disclosed that the manufacturer of the heat exchanger apparently had failed to anodize the aluminum tubes used in the heat exchanger.

... During veno-venous ECMO in a four year-old patient the platelet count was found to be below 50,000. The pediatric resident prescribed infusion of platelet concentrate. The pediatric nurse gave the platelet concentrate to the perfusionist who rapidly transfused 50 ml directly into a glass and stainless steel venous reservoir. Moments later blood in the upper one-third of the reservoir solidified into a gelatinous mass.

... In a newly established ECMO program the observation was continually being made of clot formation in the "bladder-box." After thoroughly examining their technique it was realized that the nurses were infusing hyperalimentation solution, maintenance fluid, and drugs into the ECMO circuit prior to the "bladder-box" reservoir and prior to the membrane oxygenator.

... During a trial off ECMO, the ECMO technician clamped the arterial line distal to the membrane after stopping the pump. Gas flow was not reduced and it became necessary to restore ECMO. When the clamp was removed from the arterial line and the pump was started, massive gas emboli were pumped into the patient. Investigation disclosed that the oxygenator had a pinhole leak in the membrane material, and gas had crossed into the blood side while the arterial pump was stopped.

... During a neonatal ECMO case, during periodic "flashing" of the A-V bridge, the tubing clamp on the A-V bridge was not re-applied correctly on the tubing and a large shunt existed between the arterial and venous line. The patient's condition began to rapidly deteriorate. The error was discovered before the patient expired. The ECMO was successful.

... During a routine ECMO procedure, the nurse was infusing routine maintenance IV fluid using a positive pressure infusion pump. She had either bypassed the automatic alarm or the alarm failed. Air was infused into the venous line proximal to the "bladder-box" and membrane which acted as a bubble trap. The air was aspirated and there was no apparent sequelae.

... During a neonatal ECMO case the baby's temperature fell from 37° C to 30° C within 30 minutes. The water-bath had stopped working. The unit was changed and the ECMO concluded uneventfully.

... During an ECMO case the ACTs were noted to continuously drop over several hours despite increasing heparin dosages. It was then discovered that a stopcock had been left open and the heparin had been infused onto the floor.

... During an ECMO case the PVC arterial pumphead tubing ruptured, and ECMO support was immediately discontinued while a replacement segment of tubing was inserted into the pumphead. Just prior to reestablishing ECMO, it was discovered that the tubing had been placed backwards through the pumphead. The error was corrected.

... During connection of the ECMO circuit to the patient's arterial and venous cannulae, the arterial and venous lines were reversed. The procedure commenced and the patient expired.

... On the fourth day of a nine day ECMO support the patient's right arm abruptly turned bright red while the rest of the body became cyanotic. Pump flow was reduced and cannula malposition was suspected. Venous return was normal. X-ray examination confirmed that the arterial cannula had slipped into the right subclavian artery from the aortic arch position. The physician repositioned the cannulae and the rest of the ECMO course was uneventful.

... Ten hours after beginning ECMO on a 3.6 kg baby the flow rate was 700 ml/min and the mixed venous oxygen saturation was 45% with a developing metabolic acidosis. During a routine check of the "bladder box" function, it was noted that the bladder reservoir did not collapse when the inflow line was momentarily clamped. Upon closer examination, the blood in the reservoir was seen to have settled out signifying no flow or very low flow. Slippage of roller pumphead occlusion was suspected. The patient, who was ECMO dependent, was briefly taken off support while the occlusion was reset. The occlusion locking knob had slipped. Adequate perfusion corrected the acidosis, and there were no residual problems due to the period of low flow.

... During an ECMO case false ACT results led to clotting of the entire circuit. The circuit was changed and no patient injury occurred.

Chapter 24:

CARDIOPULMONARY BYPASS IN NON-CARDIAC APPLICATIONS

Chapter 24: CARDIOPULMONARY BYPASS IN NON-CARDIAC APPLICATIONS

Cardiopulmonary bypass is being used more frequently in non-cardiac applications as perfusion teams increase in size and experience, and as non-cardiac physicians become more aware of its true potential. Early on thoracic surgeons began using cardiopulmonary bypass procedures for surgical repair of traumatic lacerations of the thoracic aorta and for surgical repair of aneurysms of the descending thoracic aorta. Cardiopulmonary bypass was also used in the surgical repair of penetrating chest wounds from knives or bullets damaging the thoracic vasculature. The bypass circuit has been used for early attempts at autotransfusion (see Chapter 21: AUTOTRANSFUSION). Extracorporeal membrane oxygenation (ECMO) is used in the treatment of the failing or injured or diseased lung (see Chapter 23: ECMO). The cardiopulmonary bypass circuit is utilized in long term support of the failing heart (see Chapter 22: CIRCULATORY SUPPORT). Many other applications have and will be utilized as the technology develops.

Perfusionists are cautioned not to be too innovative in devising circuits and using disposable equipment for purposes other than for which it was designed (see Chapter 2: LEGAL AND RISK MANAGEMENT). It is much better to use the standard cardiopulmonary bypass circuit which has stood the tried and true test of hundreds of thousands of open-heart cases and which may be a little cumbersome in special applications, but which decreases the chance of injuring a patient with a jury-rigged circuit which appears streamlined and functional but which has a not so obvious fatal flaw.

NEUROSURGERY

Neurosurgeons have and are utilizing cardiopulmonary bypass in operations on the brain.[1-4] In fact, both the early inventors of disposable extracorporeal filtration of blood were a neurologist (Swank) and a neurosurgeon (Patterson). These applications of cardiopulmonary bypass are primarily limited to surgery being performed on the cerebral vasculature for repair of aneurysms, fistulae, or injuries to the blood vessels of the brain, however hemangioblastoma resections have also been performed.[5] Cardiopulmonary bypass offers the neurosurgeon a safe and well controlled system for cooling the patient profoundly and arresting the circulation for a period of time. The neurosurgeon can then operate on arteries and veins in the brain within an essentially bloodless field. Decompression of the cerebral circulation can be accomplished, if desired, by filling the oxygenator from the superior vena caval cannula, but only if dual cannulation is used. Rewarming can then be controlled to the temperature prescribed by the surgeon. Using total cardiopulmonary bypass during the procedure removes the hazard of cardiac fibrillation during cooling and rewarming.

The patient is prepared as for open-heart surgery and the heart is cannulated in the customary manner after median sternotomy. Cooling is then accomplished per protocol (see Chapter 16: HYPOTHERMIA). Cooling should be gradual using a water-to-blood temperature of no more than 7- 10°C. Once the predetermined temperature, usually 20°C, is reached bypass should continue for a period of time until the patient has completely equilibrated to this temperature. This will normally take 20 to 30 minutes in the average adult. A tympanic or nasopharangeal temperature probe should be used since temperature variations between other measuring sites as great as 10°C have been reported.[6]

When the prescribed temperature is reached the pump is stopped and the lines are clamped. The cooler/heater unit should be turned off. It is desirable to have the capability of continuous recirculation of the contents of the oxygenator to prevent aggregation or clotting due to stasis during the period of arrest but this is not mandatory. Gas flow to the oxygenator should be reduced to 2 L/min during arrest. If recirculation of the perfusate has continued during the arrest period, it is extremely important to observe conservative temperature gradients (8°C) during rewarming since the perfusate from the oxygenator will have an extremely high pO_2. The cooler/heater unit should not be switched to the warming mode until cardiopulmonary bypass has been completely reestablished. Once the patient has been rewarmed to the prescribed temperature, the cannulae are removed and the chest is closed in the normal fashion.

Successful use of femoral vein-femoral artery cannulation and bypass in neurosurgical procedures has been reported.[5] This cannulation technique has some drawbacks in that cooling and rewarming are appreciably slower due to the flow limitations of the femoral cannulae. Presumably the neurosurgery patient has no significant cardiac disease; however, if the chest is opened, cardioplegia can be employed to protect the myocardium. This option is not available when using femoral-femoral bypass. Left heart decompression can also be effected with the open chest. With peripheral cannulation left heart distention must be monitored through a Swan Ganz catheter and if detected an apical ventricular vent is inserted by anterior thoracotomy.

VASCULAR AND CANCER SURGERY

Total cardiopulmonary bypass is used in the surgical treatment of the vascular system, particularly in the abdominal region.[7-11] The purpose of using bypass when surgery is performed in this area is to provide a means of hypothermia and circulatory arrest while having the capability of large volume autotransfusion available. The other reason for using this technique is to isolate the abdominal venous circulation.

Intra-thoracic cannulation is utilized, and the patient is cooled to the prescribed temperature. Circulation may either be stopped or continued until the surgeon determines his preference and needs. Surgical treatment may be accomplished without circulatory arrest, which is, of course, preferable. Once the surgical repair has been accomplished the patient is rewarmed, decannulated, and closed in the usual manner.

This technique is particularly useful during radical surgery of the inferior vena cava or surgical removal of neoplasms which involve that vessel. Having the patient at profound hypothermic temperatures and having the capability of instant circulatory arrest without injury to the patient may well mean the difference between life and death during an episode of massive uncontrolled bleeding. Other applications that have been reported include renal cell carcinomas which do or do not invade the inferior vena cava and operations on the renal vascular system to correct renal artery malformations and fistulae.

One method of isolating the abdominal vasculature is shown in Figure 24.1. It is possible to use this setup without a reservoir, however the incidence of sucking air in around the outflow cannulae has been reported repeatedly in the literature, and it is no longer justifiable to subject the patient to this hazard. The time or cost involved in using a collecting reservoir filled by gravity does not preclude its use. It does add a means by which volume may be withheld from the patient if necessary. It also offers access for the addition of bank blood or fluids if needed. The pump can rapidly translocate blood into the patient if needed. A large volume cardiotomy reservoir with provision for the addition of a second reservoir is the preferred system. The perfusionist should have Y connectors in various sizes along with sections of tubing in various sizes available for modification at the operative field as the pathological condition and anticipated surgical repair dictates. It is important to constantly

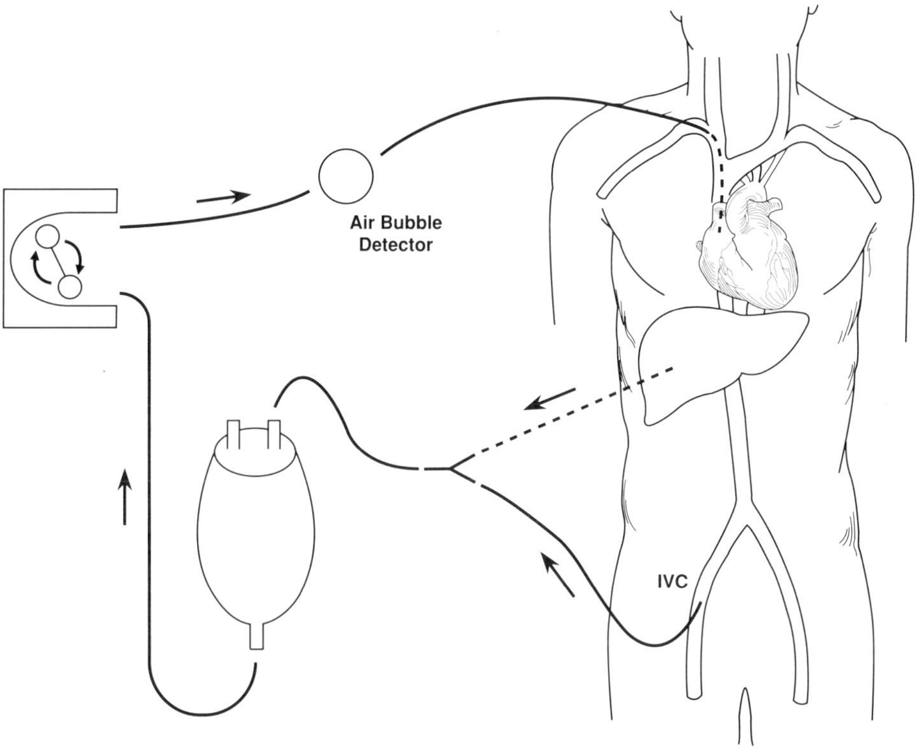

Figure 24.1 Perfusion circuit for surgery of the abdomen for operation on the inferior vena cava or other organs involving the need for vascular isolation and control. Note air bubble detector in return line. Dashed line shows second venous cannulation option if necessary to isolate operative site.

monitor both the arterial pressure and the central venous pressure in order to maintain the patient in a normal hemodynamic state during the procedure. Since cannulation is femoral-femoral in this technique, the perfusionist does not have the latitude in systemic pressure one would normally have if the patient were on total cardiopulmonary bypass.

Cardiopulmonary bypass is utilized in radical cancer surgery involving resection of the lung, esophagus and trachea. Cannulation is in the routine fashion and bypass is carried out as in open-heart surgery. Bypass allows the surgeon to more carefully resect extensive areas of lung without compromising the patient's ventilation during operation; extensive resection of the thoracic structures may be carried out with the same assurances. With proper systemic hypothermia, circulatory arrest is available to the operating surgeon. All blood suctioned from the thoracic cavity is returned to the patient. The current thinking is that cancer is in reality a systemic disease and that use of suctioned blood will not spread the malignancy.

ACCIDENTAL HYPOTHERMIA

Early and recent cases of under ice drowning and exposure hypothermia have used cardiopulmonary bypass to rewarm the victims.[12-14] Oxygenation is not the critical factor in these circumstances, but an oxygenator should be used in the circuit to control arterial pO_2 if necessary. Femoral-femoral cannulation is satisfactory in these cases. Rewarming will take a little longer due to the limitations of venous return but the reduced morbidity to the patient more than makes up for the extra time. Core warming of the internal organs should be accomplished as rapidly as is safely possible. It is vital that normal acid-base balance be maintained during rewarming. Due to the arrested circulation, metabolic acidosis will be present and may add to the myocardial irritability during rewarming resulting in fibrillation which is the primary hazard during this procedure.

Experience in resuscitation of exposure hypothermia patients using cardiopulmonary bypass for rewarming has shown that extraordinary quantitites of IV fluids are needed. It is not unusual to have to add 10-15 liters of crystalloid during the procedure. Urine output is similarly profuse.

MALIGNANT HYPERTHERMIA

Fortunately malignant hyperthermia is a rarely observed disorder, but awe-inspiring when first encountered. The disorder is pharmacologically treatable, but if it should prove refractory emergency cardiopulmonary bypass should be considered.[15] Cannulation is femoral-femoral. The bypass circuit should be primed with any solution not containing calcium (lactated Ringer's solution does contain calcium) since this element may potentiate the disorder. Cooling should be as rapid as is safe. The patient's body temperature only needs to be brought down to 36 or 37°C, so care should be taken not to over cool the patient. This is a disorder that is seen in approximately one out of 15,000 patients undergoing general anesthesia, the pediatric age group being the most common, and most often during non-cardiac surgical procedures.

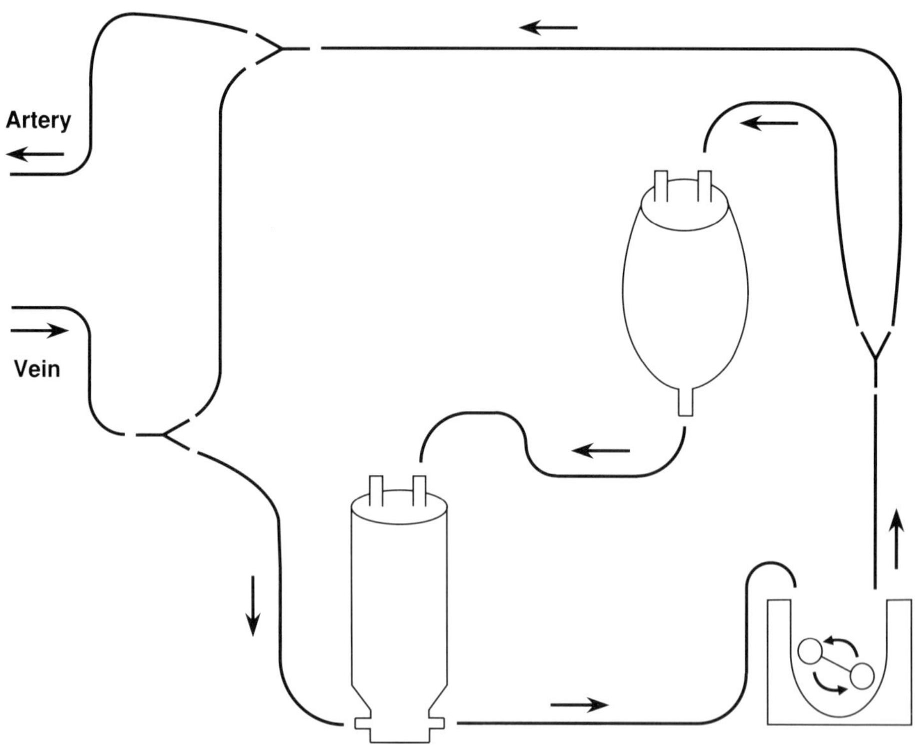

Figure 24.2 Typical perfusion circuit for chemotherapy treatment involving hyperthermia using pediatric bubble oxygenator.

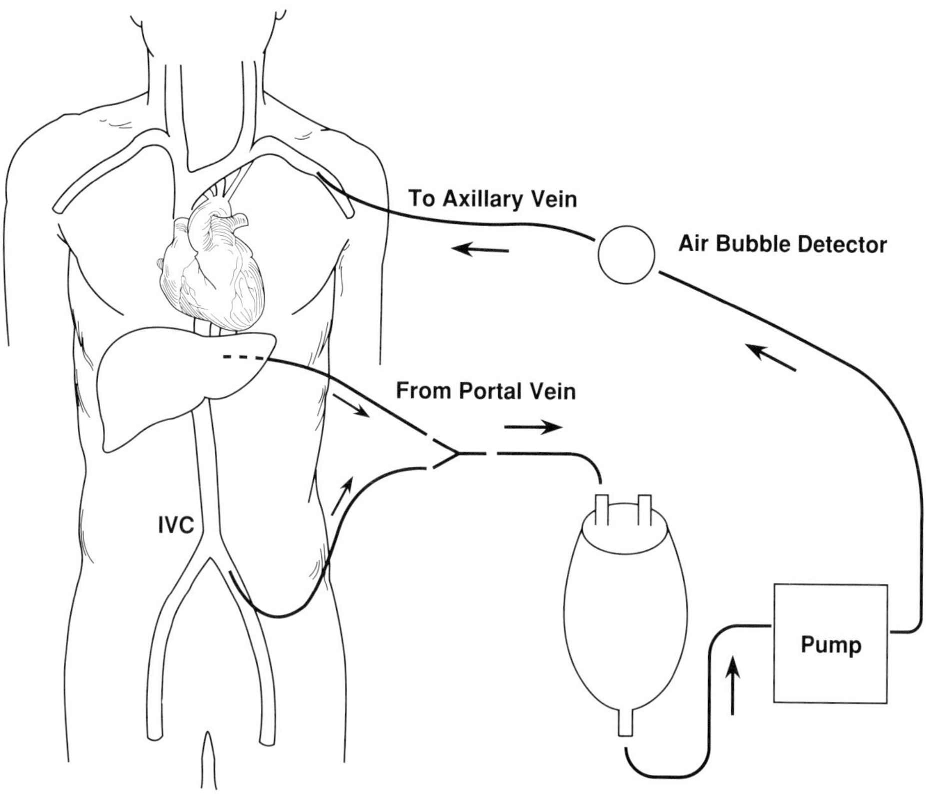

Figure 24.3 Typical perfusion circuit for liver transplantation.

ISOLATED LIMB PERFUSION AND WHOLE BODY HYPERTHERMIA

Interest in hyperthermia in the treatment of various types of cancers dates back to 1891.[15] More recent uses of hyperthermia have been in isolated limb perfusion, and most recently whole body hyperthermia[16-21] for that purpose.

Hyperthermia is effective in the treatment of certain cancers because apparently cancer cells are susceptible to elevated temperatures. Neoplasms do not vasodilate the same as normal tissue so the heat is more concentrated in the tumor.

During isolated limb perfusion additional gains are realized in reducing the toxicity and side effects of the anti-cancer drug since it is mostly removed. Cannulation is to the external iliac vessels in the leg and the axillary vessels for the arm. A pediatric oxygenator is used and primed with any suitable priming solution. Bypass is established at a flow rate of between 600 ml and 1000 ml/min. Warming is begun and when tissue sensors, placed in deep muscle, reach 40-41°C the chemotherapeutic agent is added to the perfusion circuit. Perfusion is continued for approximately one hour and then the patient is rewarmed. Fluorescine or a radioisotope is added to the perfusate to detect leakage back to the general circulation (see Figure 24.2).

In total body hyperthermia cannulation is customarily through indwelling subcutaneous grafts sutured to the femoral artery and vein. Normal femoral-femoral bypass is established and the patient is warmed to between 43-47°C. The cytotoxic agent is added to the circuit and perfusion continued at flow rates ranging from 1500 to 2000 ml/min for four hours. The treatment is usually repeated six times. A requisite of total body hyperthemia is accurate temperature sensors in both the perfusion circuit and the patient and precise control of the heat exchanger. Fluid requirements and urine output may be extraordinary during the procedure.

LIVER TRANSPLANTATION

Starzl and associates performed the first liver transplant in 1963 and the first successful liver transplant in 1967.[22] As expected, early results were less than encouraging with survival rates below 25%. As the interest and experience increased the survival rate has approached 75%. The most impressive aspect from the perfusionist's standpoint is the massive blood loss and blood usage.[23,24] Transfusions in the amounts of 251 units of red blood cells have been reported with replacement requirements due to blood loss of 2000 ml/min.

Figure 24.3 shows a typical cannulation technique for liver transplantation using heparin coated tubing and a centrifugal pump. Though expensive, the centrifugal pump is used with the reason given that the system will work without systemic heparinization. However, reports of observations of fibrin threads in the pump housing and on the struts are common. One is also cautioned not to reduce the flow below 1000 ml/min since thrombus

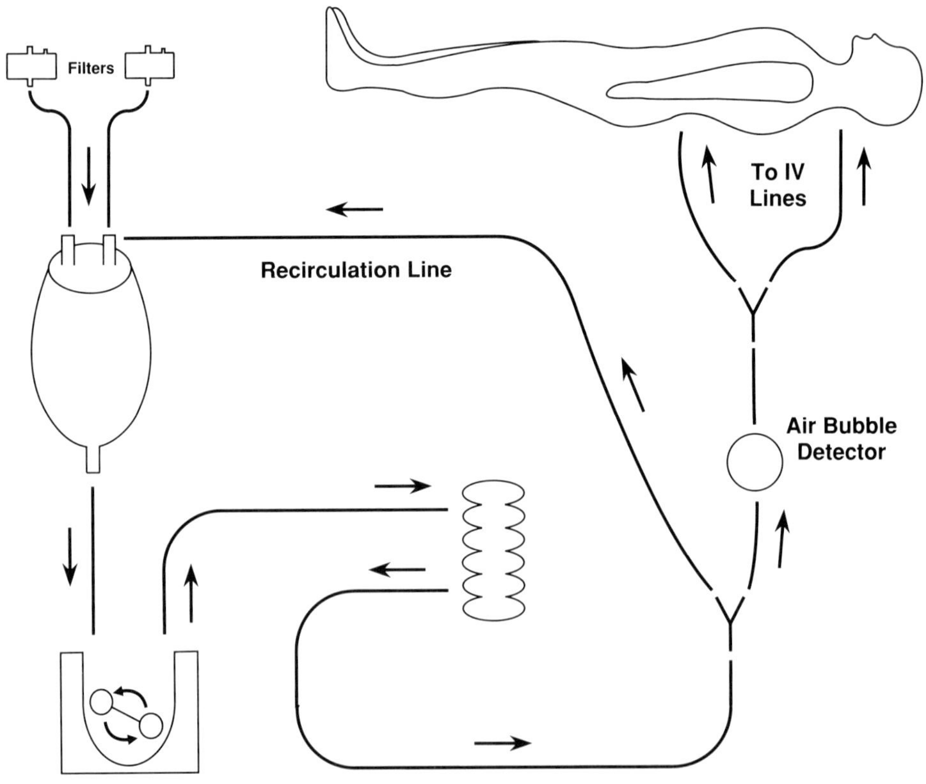

Figure 24.4 Typical rapid infusion circuit for liver transplantation or other operative techniques requiring massive rapid volume replacement. Note heat exchanger to avoid accidental hypothermia from massive fluid infusion.

formation will be accelerated in the absence of heparin. However, with the blood usage reported, one wonders how to calculate the heparin dosage if one chose to use it.

The second part of the system, the rapid transfusion system, is shown in Figure 24.4. Any massive autotransfusion system will work. One is cautioned to use two cardiotomy reservoirs and to filter the blood to 40 microns prior to admission into the cardiotomy reservoirs. It is mandatory to be able to pump from this system into the patient at a flow rate of at least 2000 ml/min. Entry is usually through two antecubital veins, but one would think that the internal jugular is a preferable route.

REPAIR OF DESCENDING THORACIC ANEURYSM

Many techniques have been employed in repairing aneurysms of the descending thoracic aorta. Those techniques include general hypothermia, internal stents and shunts, external shunts, left heart bypass, femoral-femoral bypass, and aortic occlusion proximal and distal to the aneurysm. Stents and internal shunts by design and function are the same as those used in carotid artery surgery, only larger. Externa! shunts cannulate proximal into the ascending aorta and distal either into the descending aorta distal to the aneurysm or to the femoral artery.

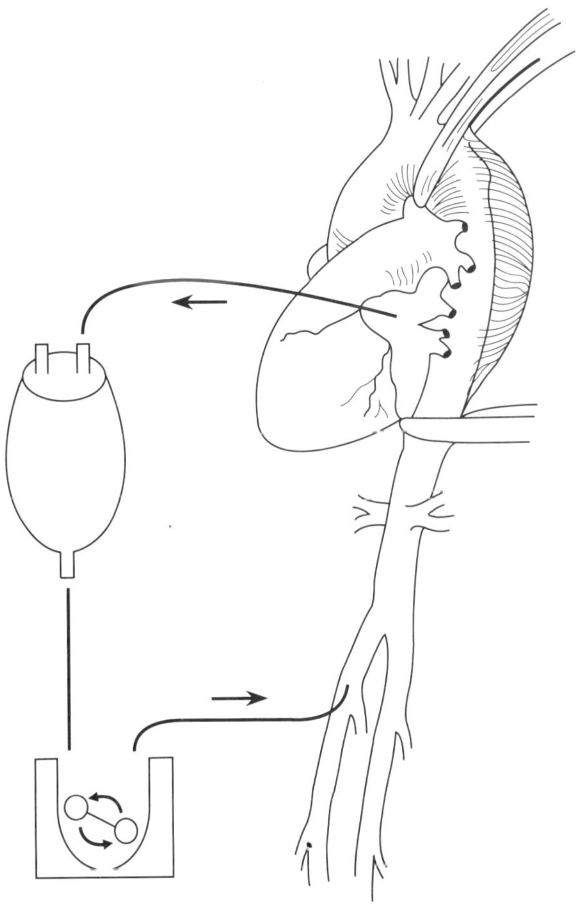

Figure 24.5 Cannulation sites used for left heart bypass and the requisite reservoir interposed between the proximal cannula and the roller pump.

Left heart bypass has been a popular method of approaching this surgical challenge. Cannulation is to the left atrium proximal and the femoral artery distally. A reservoir must be interposed between the left atrium and the roller pump to avoid generating excessive negative pressure in the left atrium (see Figure 24.5). Such an occurrence can aspirate air in around the left atrial cannula which may then be pumped out the aorta. The height of the reservoir must be constantly adjusted to control proximal systemic pressure or a clamp may be used on the return line between the left atrium and the reservoir to accomplish the same thing.

Femoral-femoral bypass using a pediatric or adult oxygenator is also a popular technique. Again, venous return must be carefully controlled either by a clamp on the venous line or by adjusting the height of the oxygenator to control proximal systemic pressure. The effect on systemic pressure is slower in response to fluid shifts than is the left heart bypass method. There may be a tendency to overshoot the desired systemic pressure in either direction. The femoral-femoral technique does provide the capability of total cardiotomy bypass if it becomes necessary.

Another technique has been described[25] in which the venous return is also controlled by a roller pump. With this technique, the arterial pump is set at an RPM to achieve a desired flow rate and the arterial reservoir level is maintained with the venous roller pump. This is an extremely accurate technique to use once the perfusionist becomes accustomed to it. The systemic pressure is usually stable within a range of approximately 200 ml in the arterial reservoir.

REFERENCES

1. Malloy KP, Hackett JE, Clark DK, Reed CC: Use of cardiopulmonary bypass, hypothermic perfusion, and circulatory arrest in the surgical management of basilar artery aneurysm. Cardiovasc Dis, Bull Tex Heart Inst 7:4, 429, 1980.
2. Woodhall B, Sealy WC, Hall KD, Floyd WL: Craniotomy under conditions of quinidine-protected cardioplegia and profound hypothermia. Ann Surg 152:37, 1960.
3. Uihlein A, Theye RA, Dawson B, Terry HR, McGoon DC, Daw EF, Kirklin JW: The use of profound hypothermia, extracorporeal circulation, and total circulatory arrest for intracranial aneurysm. Staff Meet Mayo Clin 35:567, 1960.
4. Sundt TM, Pluth JR, Gronert GA: Excision of giant basilar aneurysm under profound hypothermia. Mayo Clin Proceed 47:631, 1972.
5. Silverberg GD, Reitz BA, Ream AK: Hypothermia and cardiac arrest in the treatment of giant aneurysms of the cerebral circulation and hemangioblastoma of the medulla. J Neurosurg 55:337, 1981.
6. Silverberg GD, Reitz BA, Ream AK, Taylor G, Enzmann DR: Operative treatment of a giant cerebral aneurysm with hypothermia and circulatory arrest: Report of a case. Neurosurg 6:301, 1980.
7. Hardy DW, Reed CC, Frazier OH: The use of cardiopulmonary bypass in surgical treatment of lung cancer: Four case reports. Proceed Am Acad Cardiovasc Perfusion 2:93, 1981.
8. Deegan B, McInnis RJ, Stafford TB, Reed CC: Use of cardiopulmonary bypass for removal of an adrenal tumor and multiple pulmonary emboli: A case report. Proceed Am Acad Cardiovasc Perfusion 3:132, 1982.
9. Sadony V, Schramm G, Doetsch N: Management of extensive lesions of the lower trachea using emergency cardiopulmonary bypass. Thorac Cardiovasc Surg 27:195, 1979.
10. Hall KD, Friedman M: Extracorporeal oxygenation for induction of anesthesia in a patient with an intrathoracic tumor. Anesthesiology 42:493,1975.
11. David IB, Benak AM, Diehl JT, Goldman BS, Bruce A, Kodama R: Isolation of the retrohepatic vena cava using veno-arterial bypass with the centrifugal pump. Proceed Am Acad Cardiovasc Perfusion 7:175, 1986.
12. Davies DM, Millar EJ, Miller IA: Accidental hypothermia treated by extracorporeal blood-warming. Lancet 1:1036, 1967.
13. Truscott DG, Firor WB, Clein LJ: Accidental profound hypothermia. Arch Surg 106:216, 1973.
14. Kugelberg J, Schuller H, Berg B, Kallum B: Treatment of accidental hypothermia. Scand J Thorac Cardiovasc Surg 1:142, 1967.
15. Nauts HL, Fowler GA, Bogatko FA: A review of the influences of bacterial infections and bacterial products (Coley's toxins) on malignant tumors in man. Acta Med Scand 145(Supp) 276, 1953.
16. Frazier OH: The use of hyperthermia in the treatment of cancer. Proceed Am Acad Cardiovasc Perfusion 3:99, 1982.

17. Creech O, Krementz ET, Ryan RF, Winbland SN: Chemotherapy of cancer: Regional perfusion utilizing an extracorporeal circuit. Ann Surg 148:616, 1958.

18. McBride CM, Wilson H, Werner K, Damon F, Steinberg A: A regional chemotherapy for cancer. AmSECT Proceed 9:52 1977.

19. Stehlin HS, Giovanella BC, de Ipolyi PD, Muenz LR, Anderson R:Results of hyperthermic perfusion for melanoma of the extremities. Surg Gynecol Obstet 140:339, 1975.

20. Pettigrew RT, Galt JM, Ludgate CM, Smith AN: Clinical effects whole body hyperthermia in advanced malignancy. Br Med J 4:679, 1974.

21. Parks LC, Minaberry D, Smith DP, Neely WE: Treatment of far-advanced bronchogenic carcinoma by extracorporeally induced systemic hyperthermia. J Thorac Cardiovasc Surg 78:883, 1979.

22. Starzl TE, Iwatsuki S, Van Thiel DH, Gartner JC, Zitelli BJ, Malatack JJ, Schade BW, Hakala TR, Rosenthal JT, Porter KA:Evolution of liver transplantation. Hepatol 2:614, 1982.

23. Calder WA, Koch D, Helmrich B, Moxin J, Rhoades W: Adult liver transplantation utilizing a heparinless venous bypass system and a rapid infusion pump. Proceed Am Acad Cardiovasc Perfusion 6:81, 1985.

24. Calder WA, Hackett J:Red blood cell transfusion during liver transplantation. Proceed Am Acad Cardiovasc Perfusion 7:29, 1986.

25. Reed CC, Stafford TB: Special procedures and techniques. Ch 29 in *Cardiopulmonary Bypass*. 2nd Ed, Houston: Texas Medical Press, 1985, pp 457.

..LAWSUITS AND ...CASE NOTES

... To provide support during surgical repair of a descending thoracic aneurysm, the perfusionist devised a partial bypass circuit which included a 3/8" ID return line to a cardiotomy reservoir and a 3/8" ID perfusion line from the reservoir through a roller pump to a femoral artery cannula. The return line to the reservoir was inserted in the aorta proximal to the cross-clamp. The reservoir was only used as a collecting reservoir. During this partial bypass, flows were increased above 2 L/min. When flows were later reduced, bubbles were observed in the arterial return line. Apparently the defoaming capacity of the reservoir had been exceeded by the high flow rate and bubbles had been injected into the patient for some period of time. The patient developed an acute abdomen and was taken to surgery on the third postoperative day for exploration. At operation gangrene was observed in large areas of both the large and small bowel. The patient died from gangrene several days later.

Chapter 25:

AIR EMBOLISM

Chapter 25: AIR EMBOLISM

Apparently, Morgagni first described air embolism and investigated the entity in 1769.[1] The second patient ever to undergo open-heart surgery using total cardiopulmonary bypass suffered an arterial air embolism and expired.[2] Since this first report, every open-heart team has been plagued by this catastrophic occurrence. Because the hazard was recognized early in the genesis of open-heart surgery, many techniques and safety devices have been devised, developed, utilized, abandoned and, in some instances, retained in attempting to avoid this disaster.

Throughout this book the authors have discussed accidents involving air. Techniques have been described and, where appropriate, criticized. Hazards have been pointed out in certain accepted techniques. The safest techniques, in these authors' opinion, have been described. This chapter will deal specifically with air and its entry into the human body during open-heart surgery and cardiopulmonary bypass.

VENOUS AIR

The average paramedical person has no great respect for the infusion of air into the peripheral venous circulation and this unconcern spills over into air injected almost anywhere in the venous circulation. This thinking is dangerous and potentially lethal. The autopsy findings of a patent foramen ovale in the general population range from 25 to 50%. Thus any air introduced into a peripheral vein may have as high as a 50% chance of shunting directly into the left atrium once the air reaches the right atrium.

If the venous air reaches the lungs, the air may then enter the arterial circulation through intrapulmonary shunts, or large extra-alveolar vessels.[3,4,8] The air may also transit the pulmonary capillaries directly by the mechanism of blocking the vessel, which produces a segmental spasm, followed by relaxation and then a marked dilatation of the arterioles, capillaries, venules, and collateral channels with stasis and perivascular hemorrhage. After air is eliminated a marked increase in blood flow through the area follows which may last up to 48 hours.[5] Air can remain in the lungs a long time, long enough to cause permanent damage to the vascular beds of the lungs.[4,6]

Air can also transit the pulmonary capillary bed directly if the amount of air exceeds 0.35 ml/kg/min.[8] If air transits the heart and enters the coronary circulation, in addition to blocking blood flow in the coronary arteries, permanent myocardial damage can occur even with successful resuscitation. Air in amounts less than 0.01 ml/kg of body weight can produce irreversible damage.[7]

Because of the intermittently negative pressure in the venous circulation produced by the right heart, any puncture, tear, or opening in a vein can cause venous air embolism. One report describes a thoracotomy in which a pulmonary vein was inadvertently cut. Time to clamp occlusion was 15 seconds. The patient was declared dead 3 minutes later.[9] A 30% incidence of venous air embolism has been reported in neurosurgical patients operated upon in the sitting position.[10] One such report notes that as the muscles were being stripped from the bone an open emissary mastoid vein was noted. Simultaneously the blood pressure decreased. Through a previously placed right atrial catheter, 40 ml of air was aspirated from the right atrium.[11]

Air may also be introduced into the venous circulation by pressurizing or even introducing air into the venous return line to the oxygenator. This has been reported as happening by pressurizing the oxygenator in at least three instances.

Air has frequently been found in the left heart of drowning victims. This led to animal studies which demonstrated that, when air was forced into the trachea under a pressure of 30 mmHg, air was then found in the systemic arteries as well as the right heart of the animals.

Perhaps the most frightening study, precipitated by a venous air embolism event during insertion of an internal jugular catheter, demonstrated that, with a pressure gradient of only 4 mmHg, the flow of air through an 8 Fr cannula was 90 ml/second.[12]

CARDIOPULMONARY BYPASS AIR

Arterial Line Air

The most common source of air from the cardiopulmonary bypass circuit during bypass is from depletion of the arterial reservoir blood volume.
This can happen:

Pre or postbypass from pump-creep
Pre or postbypass from transfusion from the arterial reservoir
From inadequate debubbling of the arterial circuit
During bypass through inattention to the reservoir level
From optical illusion of blood reservoir level
From not allowing enough reaction-time-volume in arterial reservoir
By vortexing from too low an arterial blood level
From having an arterial line stopcock open
From blood clot forming in the arterial reservoir
From pressurizing an accessory Y line
From an unsecured coronary perfusion outlet
From excessive flow through an aortic cannula
From not using safety alarms
From not turning on safety alarms during bypass
From having low level safety alarm set too low on the arterial reservoir
From pressurizing the oxygenator and producing arterial or venous gas emboli
From any action that results in gas being pulled out of solution by generated negative pressure and then pumping that gas into the patient, e.g., kinked line, clamped line, etc.
From air being sucked in around the aortic cannulation site
From cracked silicone tubing in the arterial pumphead
From any cut or puncture in the arterial line
From air-lock in venous line
From oxygenator falling off bracket onto the floor
From the perfusionist being unaware that the surgeon clamped the venous line
From an inadequate tubing connection at the arterial outlet
From not using an open purge line on the arterial line filter
Using the arterial filter purge port to measure pressure
Using arterial filter purge port to sample arterial blood
Using arterial filter purge port to supply blood to hemoconcentrator or other ancillary equipment

Cardiotomy Reservoir Air

Air may originate from the cardiotomy reservoir by:

Pressurizing the reservoir and producing venous line air
Pressurizing the reservoir and producing arterial line air by pressurizing the oxygenator
Pressurizing the reservoir and producing arterial line air retrograde through an open arterial filter purge line or arterial line Y
Pressurizing the reservoir and producing arterial line air retrograde through an ancillary device blood access line to the arterial filter or arterial line Y

Membrane Oxygenator Air

This type of air may occur from:

Not adequately debubbling the bypass circuit
Not adequately debubbling the membrane
Blocking the gas outlet port while gas is flowing through a microporous membrane
Blocking the gas outlet port while gas is flowing through a non-porous membrane and rupturing the membrane
Depleting the venous reservoir bag through inattention or other reasons listed above
Air traveling down the venous line from the patient from problems with the caval cannula/ae

Vent Air

Air embolus during venting may occur by:

Vent tubing through the pumphead backwards
Vent pumphead operated in the wrong direction
Producing excessive negative pressure and pulling air out of solution
Using passive vent return to a Y connector in the cardiotomy reservoir return line can permit air to travel retrograde into the heart or aorta if the cardiotomy reservoir is pressurized or if air is allowed to travel down the cardiotomy return line from the cardiotomy reservoir
Using passive vent return to a Y connector in the venous return line can permit air to travel retrograde into the heart or aorta if an air-lock occurs in the venous line or if air returns through the venous line or if transient pressurization of the oxygenator forces oxygenating gas retrograde
Air being sucked in around the vent site
Pressurizing the cardiotomy reservoir and forcing air toward the patient past a non-occlusive vent pumphead
Using the cardioplegia cannula

Cardioplegia System Air

This can occur by:

Inattention to the cardioplegia reservoir level
Improper manipulation of a stopcock in the infusion line
A single cannula used for both infusion and venting

There may be other situations or combinations of equipment and techniques that can result in air either in the cardiopulmonary bypass system or introduced into the patient. The authors do not propose that they have listed all possibilities but only those of which they are aware.

Other Sources Of Air

These include:

Continuation of intra-aortic balloon function when the aorta is open can cause air to be sucked in through the aortotomy during deflation of the balloon
Rupture of an intra-aortic balloon in situ
Rupture of a pulsatile assist device during cardiopulmonary bypass

ANESTHETIC AIR

Typically, the open-heart surgery patient will have IV lines, an internal or external jugular line and/or peripheral venous lines for fluid and drug administration and a radial artery line for monitoring. During the procedure, temporary monitoring lines may be used in the aorta or left atrium or pulmonary artery and right atrium. Some of these may be left indwelling. It is quite easy to infuse air through these lines. If IV containers are allowed to completely empty unobserved, air remaining in the IV container may be infused. During flushing of transducers, air may be pumped into the patient through any line connected to the transducer. After bypass, if blood from the oxygenator has been transferred to empty IV or blood bags and is being infused using a pressure pump, air may be infused if the container is allowed to run dry.

The consequences of such air infusion depends upon where in the system the embolus occurs. Air introduced to the left side of the heart will probably have a more serious sequelae than air infused into the right side of the heart, but such infusion of air is not innocuous.

The anesthesiologist can inject drugs which can cause marked vasodilation resulting in an abrupt decrease in venous return. If the perfusionist is not aware or is not told of such drug administration the arterial reservoir can be depleted and air can be pumped out the arterial line to the patient.

The anesthesiologist can cause an air embolism during insertion of an internal or external jugular catheter.

OPERATIVE AIR

Cannulation

Air is usually introduced into the patient's circulatory system during cannulation of the heart.[13,31] If the aortic cannula is cross-clamped during insertion into the aorta, air bubbles from air trapped in the slanted distal tip will be forced into the aorta along with the cannula when it is inserted. The same infusion of air can occur when inserting the caval cannula/ae, which are much larger in diameter. Additionally, vena cava cannulae usually have holes in the tubing proximal to the end. If insertion is slow, air can be aspirated into the right atrium during diastole. Air is probably aspirated into the right heart during most caval cannulations. Air can also be aspirated into the right heart if the purse-string sutures are not tight around the cannula/ae or if two cannulae are inserted through the same incision or through two nearby incisions.

Vents

Insertion of a right superior pulmonary artery vent, or a left atrial vent or left ventricular vent placed via the pulmonary artery, can cause air to enter the patient in several ways. If the surgeon does not test the vent for proper operation prior to insertion, and if the vent is blowing air instead of sucking, air will be introduced into the patient's arterial system. A one-way vent valve has been available since 1964.[30] Air also may be introduced upon vent insertion in the same manner as with the aortic cannula. Also, if the vent is inserted while the heart is beating, air can be drawn into the arterial system due to pressure fluctuations (intermittent negative pressure). The air may remain resident in the pulmonary veins for a period of time or may pass rapidly through the heart.[14] The hazard to the patient's cerebral circulation is obvious when the heart is beating and the aorta is not cross-clamped.

If the vent line does not have a needle inserted in it or a vacuum relief valve, excessive negative pressure build-up in the vent line during operation can cause air to be sucked in around the insertion site. The same applies for a left atrial vent or left ventricular vent inserted through the right superior pulmonary vein. The same also applies to a left atrial vent inserted through the left atrium or a left ventricular vent inserted through the left atrium. If the negative pressure is sufficient, air may be aspirated into the pulmonary veins by a right superior pulmonary vein vent through an open aortotomy and then through the aortic and mitral valves.

This air may remain in the pulmonary veins after deairing the heart, only to be expelled later[32] (even hours later) into the coronary or cerebral arteries (see Figure 25.1). The same

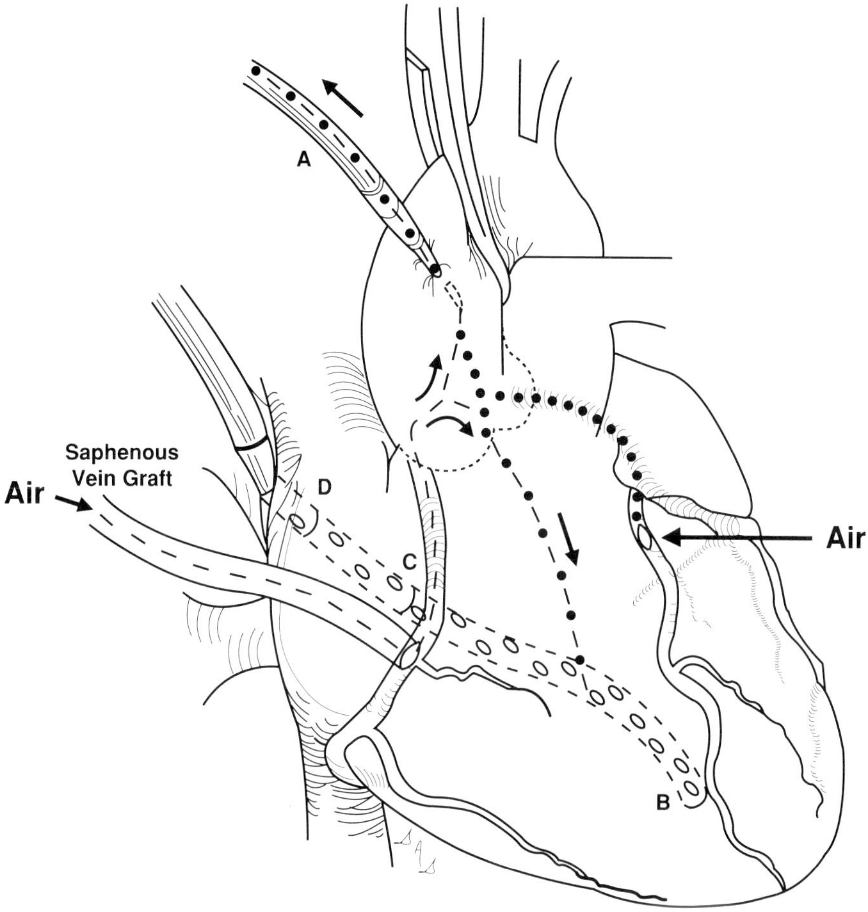

Figure 25.1 Drawing of the various left heart vent sites showing vent end positions (A is aortic root, B is left ventricle, C is left atrium, and D is right or left superior pulmonary vein). Arrows indicate possible paths of air flow retrograde from an open arteriotomy (dots) or distally anastomosed coronary graft (dashes) due to vent suction.

exact thing can occur to air aspirated around a cardioplegia infusion cannula, around an aortic vent, or from air pumped in during cardioplegia administration (the second most common cause of air embolism during bypass from the cardiopulmonary bypass circuit).

Air that enters the heart in this manner also can remain resident in the left ventricle or left atrium from inadequate deairing at the termination of bypass. Coronary or cerebral arterial air embolism is a distinct possibility from such air.

Air also may be aspirated into the heart or arterial circulation by a right superior pulmonary vein vent or a left atrial or left ventricular vent inserted via the right superior pulmonary vein through a coronary arteriotomy (see Figure 25.2), through a distally anastomosed vein graft, through a patent proximally anastomosed vein graft, through and/or around the cardioplegia cannula, and through an open aortotomy. Air may also be aspirated across a patent foramen ovale from a CVP line or internal jugular cannula.

Air aspirated into the heart or pulmonary venous circulation may cause the same problems as previously described.

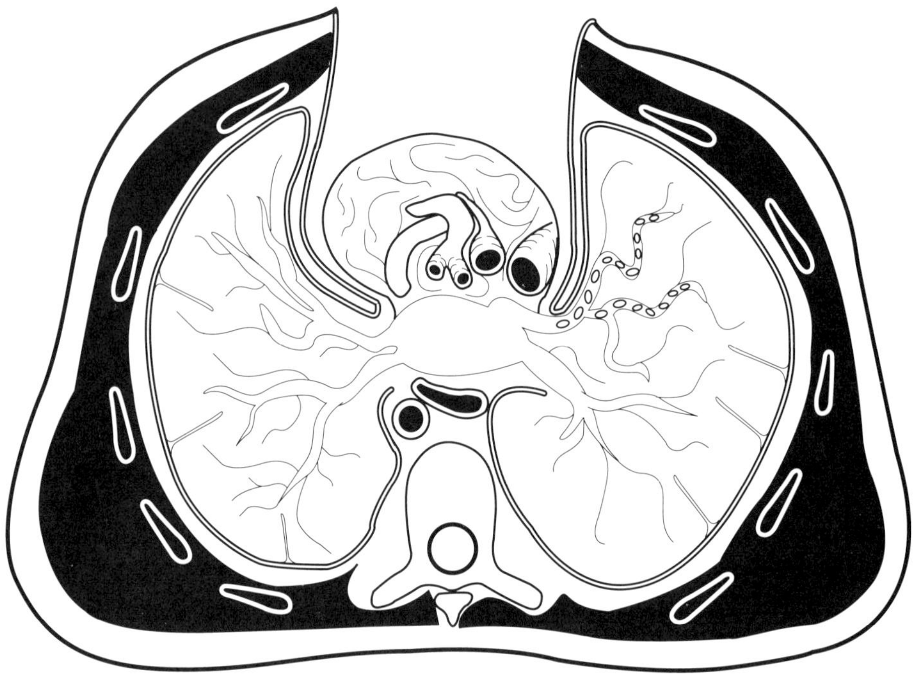

Figure 25.2 Shows the anatomical relationship of the pulmonary veins and left atrium. Air bubbles, aspirated through various sites described in the text including: right superior pulmonary vein incision, unclamped vent, aortotomy or coronary arteriotomy, are shown trapped in the right pulmonary venous system.

Venous Line

Anyone at the operative site can cause rapid depletion of the oxygenator reservoir by clamping, kinking, occluding or partially occluding the venous return line without informing the perfusionist. This can result in an empty reservoir and air being pumped into the patient through the arterial line.

The same result can occur if the caval cannula/ae slip out of the right atrium or if one or both slip out far enough for the distal side holes to pull out of the atrium.[15] Air will enter the venous line and cause a partial or complete air-lock, stopping or reducing venous return to the oxygenator. If the perfusionist does not notice, this air can be pumped through the arterial line into the patient.

Arterial Line

Air embolism can occur:

- From puncturing the arterial line with a needle, towel clamp, or other sharp object
- From using a stopcock on the connector at the aortic cannula arterial line junction which is not air tight or which is inadvertently turned the wrong way during perfusion.
- From not debubbling adequately when making the aortic cannula arterial line connection
- After the termination of bypass when the arterial pump is stopped and air, which has not been completely evacuated from the heart and aorta, rises up in the aortic cannula. This air will be pumped into the patient if transfusion from the oxygenator is resumed.

THE HEART

That air, which has entered the heart, can remain resident for great periods of time in the left ventricle, the left atrium, or the pulmonary veins has been recognized before the history of open-heart surgery recorded the first successful operative procedure.[2,14,16-20] Alexis Carrel warned of the hazard in 1914. Padula showed motion pictures of the resident air entraped in the beating left ventricle following ventriculotomy which elicited from Dr. Watts Webb the comment, "It is terrifying to realize what usually goes on in most of our patients."

After arterial line air embolism, The Survey revealed that the greatest cause of air embolism was the heart itself including: unexpected resumption of heart beat, inadequate deairing of heart, and during vent insertion and removal.

Doppler techniques for detecting intracardiac air have been available at least since 1969 when Lawrence stated, "It is our conclusions from preliminary studies that we have been 'getting away' with some things concerning air embolus that are now detectable by this technique."[21] Similar studies have described comparable techniques.[22-25]

A remarkable paper, recently published, seems to have detected, and captured on tracing, cerebral insult *at the time of occurrence* from air which had been entraped in the left ventricle when the surgeon was attempting to remove it with the aortic cross-clamp removed.[26]

The elegant study of Slogoff, Girgis, and Keats suggested that the heart and aorta were the major source of emboli causing cerebral dysfunction and consequently that arterial line filtration would not have prevented the cerebral problems.[27] Other investigators have been even more explicit. Aberg and associates state "This would point more to the operative field and the surgeon as a source of semimicroemboli than the extracorporeal equipment."[28] While Dr. Benson Roe comments succinctly, "Major cerebral air embolism during open-heart surgery is most likely to have entered the beating heart. Lesser embolic effects may occur from incomplete air evacuation or failure to divert residual air bubbles."[29]

These authors believe that the major source of air embolism during use of cardiopulmonary bypass for open-heart surgery is from within the heart and pulmonary circulation, during the operative procedure.

REFERENCES

1. Morgagni J: The seats and causes of disease. Translated from the Latin by Benjamin Alxander, London, 1769.
2. Geoghegan T, Lam CR: The mechanism of death from intracardic air and its reversibility. Ann Surg 138:351, 1953.
3. Brandes M: Ein todesfall durch emboli nach injktion von wismut salbe im in empyemafistel. Munchen Med Wchnschr 59:2392, 1912.
4. Anderson RM, Fritz JM, O'Hare JE: Pulmonary air emboli during cardiac surgery. J Thorac Cardiovasc Surg 49:440, 1959.
5. Eguchi S, Bosher LH: Myocardial dysfunction resulting from coronary air embolism. Surg 51:103, 1962.
6. Wright RR: Experimental pulmonary hypertension produced by recurrent air emboli. Med Thorac 19:231, 1962.
7. Goldfarb D, Bahnson HT: Early and late effects on the heart of small amounts of air in the coronary circulation. J Thorac Cardiovasc Surg 46:368, 1963.
8. Butler BD, Hills BA: Transpulmonary passage of venous air emboli. J Appl Physiol 59:543, 1985.
9. Chase WH: Anatomical and experimental observations on air embolism. Surg Gynecol Obstet 59:569, 1934.
10. Young ML, Smith DS, Murtagh F, Vasquez A, Levitt J: Comparison of surgical and anesthetic complications in neurosurgical patients experiencing venous air embolism in the sitting position. Neurosurg 18:157, 1986.
11. Munson ES, Paul WL, Perry JC, de Padua CB, Rhoton AL: Early detection of venous air embolism using a Swan-Ganz catheter. Anesthesiology 42:223, 1975.
12. Conahan TJ: Air embolization during percutaneous Swan Ganz catheter placement. Anesthesiology 50:360, 1979.

13. Beckman CB, Hurley F, Mammana R, Levitsky S: Risk factors for air embolization during cannulation of the ascending aorta. J Thorac Cardiovasc Surg 80:302, 1980.
14. Starr A: The mechanism and prevention of air embolism during correction of congenital cleft mitral valve. J Thorac Cardiovasc Surg 39:808, 1960.
15. Spampinato N, Stassano P, Gagliardi C, Tufano R, Iorio D: Massive air embolism during cardiopulmonary bypass: Successful treatment with hypothermia and circulatory support. Ann Throac Surg 602, 1980.
16. Willman VL, Zafiracopoulos P, Hanlon CR: Air embolism. Ch in *Extracorporeal Circulation*. Charles C. Thomas: Springfield, IL, 1958.
17. Nicks R: Arterial air embolism. Thorax 22:320, 1967.
18. Carrel A: Experimental operations on the orifices of the heart. Ann Surg 60:1, 1914.
19. Taber RE, Maraan BM, Tomatis L: Prevention of air embolism during open-heart surgery: A study of the role of trapped air in the left ventricle. Surg 68:685, 1970.
20. Padula RT, Eisenstat TE, Bronstein MH, Camishion RC: Intracardiac air following cardiotomy. J Thorac Cardiovasc Surg 62:736, 1971.
21. Javid H, Tufo HM, Najafi H, Dye WS, Hunter JA, Julian OC: Neurological abnormalities following open-heart surgery. J Thorac Cardiovasc Surg 58:502, 1969.
22. Lawrence GH, KcKay HA, Sherensky RT: Effective measures in the prevention of intraoperative aeroembolus. J Thorac Cardiovasc 62:731, 1971.
23. Oka Y, Inoue T, Hong Y, Sisto DA, Strom JA, Frater RWM:Retained intracardiac air. J Thorac Cardiovasc Surg 91:329, 1986.
24. Duff HJ, Buda AJ, Kramer R, Strauss HD, David TE, Berman ND: Detection of entrapped intracardiac air with intraoperative echocardiography. Am J Card 46:255, 1980.
25. Gallagher EG, Pearson DT: Ultrasonic identification of sources of gaseous micremboli during open heart surgery. Thorax 28:295, 1973.
26. El-Fiki M, Fish KJ: Is the EEG a useful monitor during cardiac surgery? A case report. Anesthesiology 67:575, 1987.
27. Slogoff S, Girgis KZ, Keats AS: Etiologic factors in neuropsychiatric complications associated with cardiopulmonary bypass. Anesth Analg 61:903, 1982.
28. Aberg T, Ronquist G, Tyden H, Brunnkvist S, Hultman J, Bergstrom K, Lilja A: Adverse effects on the brain in cardiac operations as assessed by biochemical, psychometric, and radiologic methods. J Thorac Cardiovasc Surg 87:99, 1984.
29. Roe B: Air embolism prevention. Ann Thorac Surg 44:212, 1987.
30. Jones RD, Cross FS: A vent valve to minimize air embolism during open-heart surgery. J Thorac Cardiovasc Surg 48:310, 1964.
31. Utley JR: Some straight thinking about venting. Course syllabus, Mechanism of Perfusion II, Tampa, Florida, 13-15 March, 1987.
32. Fishman NH, Carlsson E, Roe BB: The importance of the pulmonary veins in systemic air embolism following open-heart surgery. Surg 66:655, 1969.

..LAWSUITS AND ...CASENOTES

.. At the termination of cardiopulmonary bypass for aortic and mitral valve replacement, when the arterial pump was stopped and the arterial line clamped, air was observed to rise up in the aortic cannula. The arterial line was inspected and found to be free of air. The arterial line filter was also free of air and the purge line was open from the filter to the oxygenator. The surgeon left the operating room and informed the family that there had been an accident during operation and that the perfusionist had pumped air into the patient. The patient expired two days later.

The surviving family filed suit against the perfusionist alleging malpractice in that the perfusionist had pumped air into the patient. At trial, the jury found for the perfusionist and that no malpractice had occurred during the performance of his duties.

... On two consecutive valve patients, one mitral and one aortic, the heart was not completely deaired. When the arterial pump was stopped air rose up into the aortic cannula. The heart began ejecting when the cross-clamp was removed. Both patients expired.

.. On a mitral valve replacement procedure the heart began ejecting unexpectedly. The patient suffered permanent brain injury. Suit was filed against the surgeon. The surgeon then filed suit against the perfusionist. The case was settled out of court for an undisclosed amount.

... The surgeon was inserting a vent catheter on a redo aortocoronary bypass graft case with the aortic cross-clamp off. The beating heart sucked in air. The patient expired several days later.

... When the perfusionist was drawing a blood sample for gas analysis the surgeon inadvertently kinked the venous return line. The reservoir emptied and the pump was stopped by the air bubble detector. There was no patient injury.

... During cardiopulmonary bypass for aortocoronary bypass grafting the perfusionist allowed the oxygenator to empty. Air was pumped into the patient. The surgeon inadvertently "flashed" the cross-clamp filling the proximal aorta with air. The patient suffered moderate brain injury.

... During a total power failure and in complete darkness, the surgeon removed the cross-clamp while the heart was still open. A mixture of air and blood drained retrograde and antegrade filling the arterial line and aorta while the perfusionist was attempting to clamp the arterial line in the dark. There was no apparent injury to the patient.

... An air-lock occurred in the venous return line due to an open three way stopcock on the CVP line which filled the right heart with air. No patient injury occurred due to safety alarms.

... During total circulatory arrest, the arterial line was not clamped at the operative field or at the pump. The arterial pumphead was not occlusive and the patient exsanguinated into the oxygenator and air was aspirated into ascending aorta and aortic cannula. The air was evacuated prior to resuming bypass and no injury occurred to the patient.

... Prior to insertion of vent in a beating heart with no cross-clamp, air was aspirated into the heart and the patient subsequently expired.

... During total power failure and in darkness the perfusionist reversed the arterial pumphead while handcranking. The aorta collapsed and air was aspirated in around the aortic cannula. The perfusionist realized his mistake and started pumping in the correct direction and pumped air into the patient. The patient expired.

... The surgeon clamped the venous return line without telling the perfusionist. The arterial reservoir emptied and air was pumped into the patient. No safety devices were in use. The patient expired.

... A Swan Ganz catheter eroded into a bronchus. When ventilation was resumed, air was introduced into the left atrium and then into the arterial circulation of the patient, who expired.

... The surgeon inserted a vent into the patient while the perfusionist was out of the room. The heart was beating and the aortic cross-clamp had not been applied. The patient expired.

... An intra-aortic balloon was being used during bypass. The surgeon instructed the perfusionist to stop the pump while he reapplied a partially occluding clamp for the proximal anastomoses. The pump was stopped, the balloon deflated, and air was sucked into the aorta at the aortotomy. The patient expired.

... During cardiopulmonary bypass the perfusionist noticed a leak in the oxygenator in the defoaming area. He applied bone wax to the leak and moments later saw a massive gas embolism traverse the arterial line into the patient. The patient expired. The perfusionist had inadvertently occluded the gas exhaust holes with the bone wax and in doing so has caused pressurization of the arterial reservoir.

Chapter 26:

SAFETY AND SAFEGUARDS

Chapter 26: SAFETY AND SAFEGUARDS

Throughout this book the use of "..Lawsuits and ...Casenotes" has been utilized as practical lessons in safety and safeguards. The first section of this chapter reviews some of the important points of the preceding chapters dealing with safety as a brief synopsis.

DUTIES AND RESPONSIBILITIES

The perfusionist must be actively involved in the development of their job description and responsibilities. This is the beginning of the safe practice of perfusion. All participants in the open-heart surgery team must define their duties and responsibilities in the procedure so that everyone involved is on the same page of music and singing the same song in the same language.

LEGAL AND RISK MANAGEMENT

Modification of equipment or deviation from manufacturer's recommended procedure is a perilous practice that exposes one to unnecessary risks of posing hazards to the patient. Perfusionists must provide an acceptable standard of care in their practice of perfusion.

INTERFACE

Communication is the cornerstone to the successful outcome of an open-heart surgery procedure. Poor communication between the members of an open-heart surgery team is simply a precursor to tragedy.

CHECKLISTS

The use of checklists has been proven to be a tremendous safety factor in other similar settings, such as the aviation industry. There are just too many important details to expect anyone to remember all of them; however, **checklists are not an excuse not to think.**

CHARTING

To ask an individual to remember what occurred perhaps years in the past, to the greatest of detail, is unreasonable. Charting of events, both routine and unusual, is for the protection of the patient as well as the perfusion personnel. Properly used, charting can be a reminder of important details during cardiopulmonary bypass and the chart can function as an ongoing checklist.

BLOOD AND BLOOD HANDLING

Safety for the perfusionist in handling blood and blood products is even more important in today's operating room with the ever present risk of contracting AIDS. Patient risks are increased with each exposure to blood and blood products. Untrained perfusionists should not be involved in checking blood units.

TUBING AND CIRCUITS

As in most areas, the circuit probably should be as simple as possible and yet provide the maximum in patient care and safety. Evaluation of the circuit must be an ongoing process.

FILTRATION

These authors believe that filtration has evolved to a state where it should be used as a safety device to help decrease gross and micro gaseous emboli and debris from the extracorporeal circuit to the patient.

BLOOD PUMPS AND PULSATILE FLOW

Emergency equipment must be available on all cases and the failure of any piece of equipment must be anticipated, carefully considered and planned for.

BUBBLE OXYGENATORS

Gaseous emboli should be of prime consideration in the selection and use of a bubble oxygenator. These devices have proven their safety and efficacy of use, but must be respected for the possibility to be emptied abruptly and with little warning. The safe operation of these devices is dependant upon the experience, knowledge and diligence of the user, in conjunction with the use of available safety devices.

MEMBRANE OXYGENATORS

The safe use of membrane oxygenators is dependant upon the education and experience of the user. Each device has its own particular operating characteristics, and one must understand these differences in order to make a confident decision regarding the proper selection of a membrane oxygenator.

MONITORING DURING BYPASS

There are essential parameters that should be monitored during cardiopulmonary bypass to provide the maximum safety margin for the patient. One must appreciate the fact that most monitoring adds risk to the procedure, and one must evaluate this risk in light of the potential gain in information that might contribute to the improved care of the patient.

CONDUCT OF PERFUSION

Awareness of all activities occurring during cardiopulmonary bypass is one most important factors that contributes to a successful outcome for a patient. Concomitant with this awareness is thinking ahead and anticipating any possibility that might arise. As in high performance aircraft, the faster the plane goes, the further ahead the pilot has to think. The more complex the bypass circuit and the operative procedure, the further ahead the perfusionist must think. This important technique contributes greatly to the solution(s) necessary to provide a safe outcome to a potential accident situation resulting in an incident rather than an accident.

PEDIATRIC CONSIDERATIONS

Pediatric and infant patients are not small adult patients and cannot be treated as such. There is no substitute for experience, and this is no more glaringly apparent than in pediatric perfusion.

PERFUSION ACID-BASE BALANCE

Proper technique in using current perfusion devices should result in normal or near normal acid-base status, which is one goal of safe cardiopulmonary bypass.

HYPOTHERMIA

As an adjunctive technique, or as a routine requirement for perfusion, hypothermia requires additional thought and consideration. Water systems, heat exchangers, pressure controls, temperature monitors, and technique must be monitored and evaluated continuously. The heat exchanger/patient temperature gradient is the most important consideration in hypothermia.

PHARMACOLOGY OF BYPASS

The administration of drugs is upon prescription by a physician only. To provide maximum patient safety, perfusionists must understand the effects of pharmacology and how it affects perfusion.

MYOCARDIAL PROTECTION

The perfusionist must understand the technique and how it affects perfusion. Infusion of cardioplegia is into the aorta and demands the same respect and care as any perfusion into a patient's aorta.

EFFECT OF EXISTING PATHOLOGY

Knowledge of pathology is necessary in order to evaluate its effect on cardiopulmonary bypass. Some conditions can have deleterious effects on the perfusion and therefore patient safety.

EFFECT OF SURGICAL TECHNIQUE

In order to provide maximum safety for a patient undergoing cardiopulmonary bypass, the perfusionist must be prepared for the unusual and unexpected that may become an eventuality during any open-heart procedure. There is no substitute for education, experience, pre-planning, and effective communication.

AUTOTRANSFUSION

Air embolus is a definite hazard associated with autotransfusion. The autotransfusion unit **should never be pressurized** during operation, and the recovered fluid should be filtered and reinfused by a volume controlled pump.

CIRCULATORY SUPPORT

Additional equipment used during cardiopulmonary bypass should be operated by additional personnel and must not detract from the primary responsibility of the perfusionist.

ECMO CIRCUITS AND TECHNIQUES

The longer that a patient is perfused or supported, the more exposure that patient has to risks. Anticoagulation, flow control, venous return, temperature, sterility, and the length of the procedure are of prime concern.

CARDIOPULMONARY BYPASS IN NON-CARDIAC APPLICATIONS

These procedures require more forethought, planning, and ingenuity than routine open-heart total bypass procedures to provide maximum patient safety.

AIR EMBOLISM

The introduction of air into the cardiovascular system is the single most profound hazard to patients undergoing cardiopulmonary bypass. Attention to detail, especially the level in the oxygenator reservoir, must be the most important concern of the perfusionist.

SPECIAL SAFETY DEVICES

Safety devices have been used and described long before the first sucessful clinical cardiopulmonary bypass procedure.[1,2] Gibbon described a level sensor in 1937 and Clark and Gollan had used one in the laboratory, reporting the results in 1952. Both devices involved feedback circuits to the pump RPM control. Effler reported the clinical use of such a device in 1958.[3] It is unfortunate that the development of safety devices through the years did not meet the expectations and visions of the early investigators nor keep pace with the requirements of the perfusion profession. Even more regrettable is the resistance to acceptance and use of safety devices by some small sector of perfusionists.

Patient Safety Devices

There are no devices known by these authors that are attached to, or that are inserted into, the patient that are used as safety devices. There are many devices used for monitoring, or to provide data for decision making, but not as direct safety devices to protect the patient.

Venous Circuit Devices

There are no devices known to these authors that are placed in the venous circuit and are direct safety devices for the protection of the patient.

Cardiotomy Circuit Devices

With the exception of extracorporeal filters available to insert into the circuit, or those filters that are integral in some cardiotomy reservoirs, there are few devices available. Those filters inserted into the cardiotomy return line to the oxygenator provide a measure of gaseous emboli protection from the small bubbles generated by the cardiotomy suction system. However, the proper use of the cardiotomy reservoir will provide additional protection.

One-way valves are available for insertion into the vent line to prevent air from being infused retrograde from the vent pump into the heart as well as prohibiting excessive negative pressure generation. These lines must be checked prior to use because there have been reports of these valves being inserted into the line backwards.

Arterial Circuit Devices

A properly used arterial line filter should be considered a safety device in the arterial circuit. Most perfusionists, 88% of respondents, used an arterial filter as a bubble trap. In order to function as a bubble trap, a filter in the arterial line must be continuously vented to a low pressure or no pressure site in the bypass circuit. This purge must never be interrupted in order to prevent gas from crossing the filter media should a significant amount of gas enter the inlet of the filter. **If the arterial line filter is not constantly and properly purged it is not a safety device and will not perform a safety device function.**

There are one-way valves available for use in the arterial purge line that keep air from going retrograde from the purge to the filter. Stopcocks should not be used on the purge outlet of the filter.

There is still available gross air bubble traps that were used in the past to add a measure of protection or safety in the arterial line. These bubble traps do not appear to be as effective as an arterial line extracorporeal blood filter in removing micro air from the system, and their efficiency in removing gross air has not been established.

Some arterial pressure monitors have alarms on them that can be set to most any pressure limit and give an audible and/or visual alarm if this limit is exceeded.

Low level alarms are available either integral to the heart-lung machine or as ancillary devices. Most integral alarms have the added safety benefit of being able to stop, at least, the arterial pumphead if the alarm is triggered. Ancillary devices do not generally perform this automatic function. Both types of devices are dependent upon the perfusionist turning on the alarm sensor and secondly at what reservoir level the perfusionist has placed the sensor on the oxygenator.

Arterial line bubble detectors detect gas bubbles in the arterial line. The limitation is usually a bubble which is one ml in volume. These devices can automatically stop the arterial pumphead if a gas bubble is detected. The same limitations apply as to low level sensors. The perfusionist must turn on the device for it to function. The device should be installed on the arterial line distal to the oxygenator and proximal to the arterial pumphead.

It is the position of these authors that at least two of the available safety devices in the arterial circuit must be used on every cardiopulmonary bypass procedure.

EDUCATION

Probably the single most important safety factor in perfusion is education. Education comes to the perfusionist in many shapes, forms and sizes. Of course, formal education is important for a proper base to enable one to start their pursuit of a true educational experience. Education truly commences when someone graduates from perfusion school and begins their career.

As one gains experience in perfusion one begins to realize that their education, experience, and growth is a continuing process. The most successful perfusionists realize that they learn everyday, and that they learn from many different sources. This could be considered as consultative education. It may come from formal professional meetings, from small informal group meetings, or just from individual discussions with associates or colleagues. It may come from reading and reflection. The source of knowledge is not important, the pursuit of knowledge is.

Another important point in education is understanding. A dedicated perfusionist will continually seek the answer to the most important question: Why? The world has been a better place because individuals in all walks of life have searched for the answer to this question. And absent the answer, acceptance. If one understands why something is the way it is, or why something occurred, they have begun the journey down the path in pursuit of excellence. This path may, providentially, have no end.

CONCLUSION

Throughout this book the authors have dedicated most of the space to safety involving cardiopulmonary bypass equipment. Because this is a text about technique, it has been most important to emphasize the *safe techniques* that should increase the capability of producing favorable results or outcomes for patients undergoing this most demanding technical procedure.

The most important safety device in the cardiopulmonary bypass circuit is the perfusionist. It does not have to be turned on, or placed in the right location. It does not short out or run away or creep or experience power failure. The only requirement is that it fully utilize its brain.

The perfusionist is the redundant safety backup system of all available safety devices with their limitations and failings. The perfusionist is also the first line safety device. There were safety devices after there were perfusionists, this resulting from the fact that perfusionists are human beings with inherent limitations and failings. Thus there is and must be an interaction between the perfusionist and the safety devices. They compliment each other and provide overlapping coverage of the deficiencies of each.

Safety is an attitude.

It is an approach to a process that involves dedication to detail, commitment to excellence, and uncompromising respect for human life and sovereignty. Each of these principles are difficult, if not impossible, to teach someone in the course of a technical education process. Society, in general, in this country has undergone some very interesting changes since the early 1960s. Most of these changes involve or affect some of the attitudes toward the principles described. These changes in social attitudes, of course, affect change in the health care profession as a whole, which comprises only a small part of society. During this same time period, there has also been a period of tremendous growth in the perfusion profession. So it perhaps has to be expected that these changes may have had a greater impact on this profession than in others of our society.

Dorland's Medical Dictionary does not contain the word "safety," nor "safe," or "safeguards." It does describe "perfusion" which is perhaps a medical testimony of how technological development can speed past human development.

There have been many psychological and social studies that demonstrate, in the human subject, that the more involved people become with technical development, the less compassionate and concerned about human development they become. This is described as "High Tech / Low Touch." It simply means that the tremendous technical revolution that has touched every area of society, and especially perfusion, has left all of us somewhat less concerned about the humanitarian side of our development than we are about technical achievement. There is no question about the quality and success of the technical evolution of the equipment, and people that operate that equipment. There is room for question about our human development.

Safety is a committed respect for the human lives in which we have a responsiblity.

In the confusion of today's medical world the general public is anxious about the health care system. A climate of distrust of everyone in the health care profession has resulted in many social dilemmas that involve attitudes toward safety in the operating room and even the fear of making important difficult decisions that may change many peoples lives forever.

It is not the purpose of these authors to produce fear of decision making, or to cause any threat in any way to the ongoing development of perfusion techniques. In the thirty years of evolution of the techniques used for perfusion there has not been a text written to encompass the responsibilities of a perfusionist. It is important in such a text to emphasize over and over that the most important technique involved in perfusion is safety.

The authors realize and appreciate that to develop a totally and completely "safe" perfusion system would require a financial commitment at least equal to that enjoyed by the space shuttle program. This does not alter their commitment to the profession nor detract from their pursuit of the "safe" system. The authors further realize and appreciate the fact that the most important safety feature of the bypass system today is the perfusionist. This does not alter their concern about the commitment of the profession to excellence, or their obligation to help develop attitudes of commitment to excellence.

It appears that the general prime motivation for entrance into the perfusion field today does not involve visions of commitment or compassion for fellow human beings, but perhaps those 1960s values of money and social status. No matter what the attitude of today's professional perfusionists might be, before there will be a "safe" system there must be a total commitment to an attitude of safety and a total respect for the individuals that trust us with their only valuable possession ... their very lives.

REFERENCES

1. Gibbon JH: Artificial maintence of circulation during experimental occlusion of pulmonary artery. Arch Surg 34:1105, 1937.
2. Clark Jr LC, Hooven F, Gollan F: Large capacity, all glass oxygenator and pump. Rev Sci Instrument 23:748, 1952.
3. Olmsted F, Kolff WJ, Effler DB: Three safety devices for the heart-lung machine. Cleveland Clin Quart 25:169, 1958.

Index